Supernormal

*Science, Yoga, and the
Evidence for Extraordinary
Psychic Abilities*

Supernormal

DEAN RADIN, PhD

DEEPAK
CHOPRA
BOOKS

Published in the United States by Deepak Chopra Books, an imprint of the Crown
Publishing Group, a division of Random House, Inc., New York.

www.crownpublishing.com

DEEPAK CHOPRA BOOKS and colophon are trademarks of Random House, Inc.

Library of Congress Cataloging-in-Publication data is available upon request.

ISBN 978-0-307-98690-0
eISBN 978-0-307-98691-7

Printed in the United States of America

Cover design by Nupoor Gordon
Cover illustration: © NLD/Shutterstock

10 9 8 7 6 5 4 3 2 1

First Edition

To Susie and to my parents,
Hilda and Jerry Radin

CONTENTS

CONTENTS

PART III: *. . . And Beyond*

BY DEEPAK CHOPRA

Foreword

The strange thing about the paranormal—or the supernatural, the miraculous, and all other synonyms—is that no matter how often you prove it, it remains unproven. There have been hundreds of studies on clairvoyance and viewing at a distance, arising from age-old experience. Invariably, as Dean Radin patiently explains in this book, the experiments indicate that the experience of reading someone else's thoughts, seeing a faraway event, or anticipating the future is real. Ever since science demolished faith as a way of knowing reality, facts are supposedly supreme, and when the same fact is repeatedly shown to be true, that is enough to change accepted reality. So why, in this case, have facts proved helpless?

The answer is complex, subtle, and yet as common as any ingrained prejudice. Facts don't change minds as often as they confirm what the mind insists on believing. Therefore, the path from faith to facts is much more fragile than we like to think, and along the way are crouching adversaries—hidebound beliefs, stubborn biases, ad hominem attackers, skeptics who know in advance that X cannot be true, and the most elusive of adversaries, collective consciousness. Mass opinion can stop an unwelcome fact in its tracks, which has happened for centuries when miracles, wonders, magic, and the paranormal have been too uncomfortable to confront. Behind the cliché that you create your own reality there is a shadow: If you don't create your own reality, it will be created for you.

For this reason, Radin's discussion of supernormal abilities, which were first explained in a systematic way in an ancient Indian text known as the *Yoga Sutras* of Patanjali, walks a double line. He presents the amassed evidence for all kinds of "superpowers" while nudging us persuasively to look at why something can be proven and unproven at the same time. This double track is the only sensible way to get people to change their minds, adhering to the familiar adage "A man convinced against his will is of the same opinion still." Any number of controlled studies have demonstrated that when people are presented with facts that contradict their firmly held beliefs, they tend to ignore the facts; even more perversely, a sizable percentage of people will become more confirmed in their beliefs the more contravening facts you present.

The grassroots spiritual movement tagged generically as the New Age firmly divided society into believers and nonbelievers in all kinds of matters that Radin covers, and he is mature in approaching hot-button topics as a peacemaker, not another divisive voice. That's a fortunate stance. When science already has ample evidence about phenomena that are firmly excluded from the official picture of reality, winning acceptance requires a grasp of human psychology. The art of persuasion is subtle, but it is also based on everyday experience:

> Why prove to a man he is wrong? You can't win an argument, because if you lose, you lose it; and if you win, you lose it. You will feel fine. But what about him? You have made him feel inferior, you hurt his pride, insult his intelligence, his judgment, and his self-respect.

This piece of practical psychology, written decades ago by Dale Carnegie, becomes relevant to the paranormal once you substitute the word *scientist* for *man* in the first sentence. The reason that facts are secondary in proving the validity of superpowers is that science, like any human enterprise, is overseen by individuals who have a stake in what they do, and that stake includes pride, intelligence, judgment, and self-respect, as Carnegie grasped.

In *Supernormal*, Radin calms our nerves and our prejudices at the same time, which levels the field. He is willing to call the path of yoga, which is held to develop supernatural abilities, "legendary," but he also fixes his stern gaze on science's self-contradiction when it refuses to accept findings that were arrived at through impeccable use of the scientific method. As he wryly notes, if science is to change in the direction of a new reality, teeth grinding has to lessen over time.

But why a new reality and what does it have to do with levitation, clairvoyance, invisibility, and many other claims that Patanjali made? The simple answer is that the old reality has worn itself out. In a chapter devoted to the Eightfold Path of Science (a play on the Eightfold Path of Buddhism), Radin looks at the principles that modern science is based upon and shows, quite accurately, that many were exploded by the quantum revolution a hundred years ago, and others have been steadily weakened. Once time and space were no longer absolutes, once physical objects were reduced to whirling clouds of energy and cause and effect turned into a game of probabilities instead of certainties, there was a radical shift in how reality is perceived.

This shift is amazingly consonant with the ancient seers of India, and for forty years quantum concepts have been woven into spiritual concepts, with voices ranging from a physicist like Fritjof Capra to a spiritual luminary like the Dalai Lama confirming the parallels. Radin adds his voice to a veritable chorus but with restraint. His talent lies in returning to basics and finding common ground. Well aware that few people outside the specialized field of ancient Indian studies will know of the *Yoga Sutras*, and who will blink to see Sanskrit terms like "siddhi" and "samyama," he travels adeptly between common experience (especially psi experiences of clairvoyance and subtle intuition) and the arcane of mysticism. The goal is to persuade the reader, not against his (or her) will but with willing cooperation. "Remember when X happened to you? Well, the same thing was known to the seers of yoga and has been shown to be valid in the laboratory."

Radin's aim isn't to make his own version of reality the right one. Instead, he wants to show that there are more choices than people generally realize, and some of those choices add greater power to the mind, increase the potential for uncovering greater insight, and eventually turn the cliché of "You can create your own reality" into a living experience. Radin doesn't proselytize about which version of reality anyone should choose, but in his evenhanded way he is also insistent that some realities that seem outlandish to science, such as the reality where a person can levitate, are not ridiculous, superstitious, or ignorant. Hundreds of observers have recorded in private diaries, public statements, and sworn oaths that they saw Joseph of Cupertino levitate (among the many levitating Catholic saints, this seventeenth-century figure was alive almost fifty years after the death of Shakespeare), and Radin makes note of it without apology or second-guessing.

Yet this book isn't a wonder-working checklist from the past. It goes beyond the worldview in which miracles are unquestioned and the opposing worldview, in which miracles are preposterous, to find reconciliation. To some extent, the judgment of Solomon is involved—both sides have something to say and something to learn from each other. (Reconciliation was on Einstein's mind when he made his famous comment, "Science without religion is lame, religion without science is blind.") Clearly that's not good enough, because reality stares us in the face, and we must relate to its actuality. Endless arguments over how to model reality—for science and religion are merely models—are digressions.

With that in mind, Radin doesn't lose sight of the radical mystery that reality poses, not just to mystics but to hard-nosed realists among the quantum pioneers. In the book's closing pages, two stark statements of fact are quoted. The first comes from Max Planck, who originated the quantum revolution:

I regard consciousness as fundamental. I regard matter as derivative from consciousness. We cannot get behind consciousness. Everything that we talk about, everything that we regard as existing, postulates consciousness.

Planck felt that he was stating a fact that couldn't be evaded (which turned out to be a poor prediction of how powerful evasion can be). Since Patanjali and all the Vedic seers espoused consciousness-based reality, Radin has subtly turned the tables. It's not yoga's job to prove that consciousness is the foundation of all experience; it's science's job to prove that it isn't. Such proof is far from forthcoming. But Radin optimistically points out that a new generation of scientists, less liable to grind their teeth, is steadily coming to terms with consciousness as a factor that cannot be set aside, evaded, wished away, or treated with contempt.

To support his optimism, Radin quotes another quantum pioneer, Wolfgang Pauli: "It is my personal opinion that in the science of the future reality will neither be 'psychic' nor 'physical' but somehow both and somehow neither." In other words, the issue is not either/or, but both/and, a point that this book emphatically declares. To take consciousness seriously is a step in the evolution of science, one that extends the "spooky" nature of the quantum world. Spookiness isn't going away; neither are the world's wisdom traditions. Two camps of visionaries, from the distant past and the fringes of the present, are advancing on us. Their message is about the conscious evolution of humanity, and as this perceptive book shows, when the two camps of visionaries merge, nothing will ever be the same.

Preface

All of man's problems come from his inability to sit
quietly in a room alone.

—*Blaise Pascal*

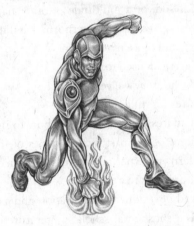

It took a while to scramble out of the mud. Then, in a flash of ga-
lactic time, we've built magnificent cities and civilizations, flown to
the moon and back, and landed robots on Mars. Are such feats the
pinnacle of humanity, the very best that we can hope to achieve? Or
can we imagine even more astonishing futures? Is it possible that the
superpowers described in ancient legends, science fiction, and comic
books are patiently waiting for us behind the scenes, poised for an evolutionary twitch to pull the trigger?

Similar questions have been asked by visionaries throughout history, and many techniques have been developed to explore and develop our potentials. One of the most effective methods is also one of the most ancient—yoga.

The word *yoga* is a cognate of *yoke*, meaning "to combine, connect, or unify." What is said to be unified is the personal self and the universal Self. This rarified state is a goal of nearly all esoteric practices. It is also known as achieving a state of *illumination*, or to be *awakened* or *enlightened*. The shift from everyday awareness to an ecstatic form of consciousness gives one direct access to knowledge of unmediated Reality. From that place one finds that personal awareness becomes aligned with or is absorbed into a universal Mind, Divine Consciousness, Great Spirit, God, or a multitude of other names used for the transcendent. It also gives rise to supernormal abilities, with "powers and abilities far beyond those of mortal men!" as the narrator from the 1950s TV show *Superman* used to say.

At least, that's the story we've been told by yogis, sages, and mystics from all cultures for millennia.

The question addressed in this book is how to interpret such fantastic claims in light of the past five centuries of scientific advancement. In the modern era, especially within Western culture, claims of enlightenment or union with a universal Self span a spectrum of belief ranging from awed devotion to exasperation and anger at New Age twaddle. There is a substantial scholarly literature on the formative role of mysticism, miracles, and claims of the supernormal in religion, but most scientists (and surprisingly, most scholars of comparative religion) have been taught to consider supernormal capacities as an embarrassment of medieval times, and as such not worthy of serious attention.

The term "supernormal" was coined by the British classicist Frederic Myers, one of the founders of the (London-based) Society for Psychical Research in 1882. Myers used this word to refer to natural, lawful phenomena that presaged a more advanced, future stage of human evolution. Such phenomena, including psychic abilities like clairvoyance, may be regarded today as anomalous or as unbelievable. But in the future, according to Myers's conception, as we gain an improved understanding of ourselves, our capacities, and the physical world, the supernormal will become completely normal.

Has our sophisticated scientific understanding of reality developed blinders when it comes to reports of the supernormal? Could it be that when the blinders are removed, there actually is something interesting going on? Are *all* reports of mystical or psychic experiences, of communion with realities that transcend the mundane, necessarily mistaken?

This question is motivated by more than simple curiosity. We know that reports of such experiences have not faded away with the stellar rise of science. Many people today still believe in miracles and psychic phenomena. They believe not because of stories they've heard, or because of unquestioned faith, but because of firsthand personal experience. A Harris poll in 2009 found that a whopping 76 percent of Americans believe in miracles. A CBS News poll conducted the same year found that 57 percent of Americans believe in one or more psychic phenomena. This majority includes well-educated academics and scientists, some of whom are experts in the frailties and biases of the human psyche.

We now know that glib explanations of these beliefs offered by skeptics, that they are due solely to misfirings of the brain, or to various cognitive or educational defects, are simply wrong. A growing body of scientific evidence indicates that some experiences labeled psychic are not illusions or delusions—they are genuine cases where "superpowers" of consciousness occur, often spontaneously.

Remarkably few scientists have paid attention to this evidence. And yet the people who report these experiences rank them as among the most profound and transformative events in their entire lives. One would think that this fact alone would attract a little attention.

Beyond questions of personal interest, many of the sages and geniuses responsible for shaping civilization as we know it today wrote about the influence of exalted states of intuitive awareness on their actions. This means that our understanding of transcendent experience goes beyond mere academic interest—it goes to the very heart of the perennial questions that have captured the attention of anyone who has ever wondered, "Who am I?," "Why am I here?," and "What's it all about?"

Without acquiescing to the social pressure in science that encourages a careless dismissal of the evidence, we will also avoid collapsing into an uncritical, starry-eyed acceptance of all purported miracles. The approach we'll take is to examine one of the better known transformative paths—yoga—to see if any of the guideposts to enlightenment in that tradition have been scientifically confirmed. If it turns out that there are rational reasons to accept *any* of the claims of supernormal abilities, even one, even a tiny smidgeon, then perhaps the mystics were not just spinning tall tales and we would be justified in reconsidering ancient wisdom on these matters.

This topic is not for everyone. Some people have neither the disposition nor the patience to seriously consider phenomena that are not overwhelmingly self-evident. As Woody Allen once quipped, "I'm astounded by people who want to 'know' the universe when it's hard enough to find your way around Chinatown." Then there are those at the other end of the spectrum, including some yoga devotees, who accept the legendary superpowers described in ancient texts on faith alone. For them scientific arguments are tedious and irrelevant.

But as long as these questions can be asked, some fraction of the population will be motivated to look beyond dogma pro or dogma con. This is a good thing, because history teaches us that some portions of today's scientific worldview, that set of theories about who we are, what we're capable of, and the nature of reality, are wrong. The same is equally true for some portion of our religious and spiritual beliefs. We don't know yet exactly where we've got it wrong, but if there's any chance of humanity evolving out of its rough adolescence, then we must correct our misunderstandings, and soon. What we'll explore in this book is the possibility that legends about yoga superpowers can provide hints about how we might do this, or at least how we might reconsider the scope of human potential.

We are at the threshold of gaining new answers about the legendary superpowers. What we'll find is that it's now possible to state with confidence that *some* key elements of stories about the yoga superpowers are true, and as a result there is some scientific support for the ontological reality of the mystical realities underlying most religions. The universe, and our role in it, is beginning to look more interesting than our textbooks have led us to believe, even after taking into account all the astonishing discoveries science has found so far.

· · ·

In previous books, I've mentioned similarities between ancient stories of mystic powers and several common psychic phenomena, including telepathy and precognition. I mentioned how these abilities, known as the *siddhis* (pronounced sid-hees), are associated with the intense meditation practices of advanced yoga.[1, 2] Partially because of my interest in this topic, I was invited by the Indian Council for Philosophical Research to be its National Visiting Professor for 2010. I traveled throughout India under the auspices of this Indian government-sponsored program, and I gave a series of talks about science and the siddhis at traditional universities and at universities specializing in the study and practice of yoga and ayurvedic medicine. In India, both types of universities carry the same academic status when sanctioned by the government.

I noticed that the yoga siddhis, a subset of which Westerners would call psychic phenomena, are so well integrated into Indian culture that hardly anyone there bothers to study them scientifically. Psychic effects are considered ho-hum supernormal abilities that some yogis and *sadhus* (holy men) possess. They are understood as refined aspects of mind and consciousness that have been discussed in great depth by scholars and practitioners for millennia.[3, 4] Why bother studying something with the newfangled tools of science when it is already accepted as commonplace?

By contrast, in the West the mere existence of psychic phenomena remains a contentious issue, despite persistent interest and popular belief. There are a number of reasons for this chronic tension. On the religious side, within the Judeo-Christian-Islamic traditions, only God (or those he appoints) is allowed to perform miracles. Ordinary folks who perform such feats are considered suspect (by theists) if they're lucky and heretical if they're not. And on the scientific side, there is a widely held (but incorrect, as we'll see) assumption that these phenomena cannot exist because they violate one or more scientific principles.

Most scientists haven't had the audacity to publicly challenge that assumption; it's too dangerous to swim against the tide. But the stigma of the woo-woo taboo hasn't been sufficient to override everyone's curiosity about phenomena at the edge of the known. And as a result, the irony is that the skeptical West has learned more about the scientific evidence for the siddhis than the sympathetic East.

• • •

Before we begin, three notes for the reader. The first is about diacritical marks. Some of the terms I use are from the ancient Indo-Aryan language, Sanskrit. There is a traditional elegant script for Sanskrit called Devanagari. In modern times a transliteration method for Sanskrit, based on Roman letters, is used to indicate proper pronunciation. That scheme uses a wide range of diacritical marks. For example, "Yoga Sutras" may be written as *Yoga-Sūtras*, "Sankhya" philosophy as *Sānkhya*, or "samadhi" as *samādhi*. These markings denote nuances in tone and emphasis, but I've found that for native English readers these notations also tend to be distracting, so in this book I don't use them. I trust that the meaning of the words will still be clear.

The second note is that while I focus on a classic yoga text—Patanjali's *Yoga Sutras*—as a convenient historical road map for discussing supernormal abilities, I occasionally refer to other mystical and religious traditions. I do this not because yoga and, say, Tibetan Buddhism, are interchangeable (although discussion of superpowers was an important part of early Buddhism[5]), but because occasionally it is more convenient to make a point with a story from one tradition rather than another. I justify this casual hopping among traditions because we are interested in broad-brush similarities, and because our main interest is the scientific evidence for supernormal abilities rather than the refined discernments one expects from scholarship in comparative religion.

Finally, at the back of the book there are several pages of notes that may clarify certain technical points.

So I apologize to purists who may be annoyed by my lack of attention to the philology of Sanskrit and to my simplification of an immensely rich ethnohistorical and religious literature.

Supernormal

PART I

From Legendary Yoga Superpowers . . .

In a world before the Internet, before smartphones and energy drinks, there were legends of superpowers: Seeing hidden objects and distant events. Knowing the future. Walking on water. Instant healing.

Such legends are still vibrantly alive. They are staple themes in science fiction and permeate the entertainment industry. The majority of the world's population believes in one or more of them. They are presented as fundamental truths in most religions. They've gained labels such as telepathy, clairvoyance, precognition, and psychokinesis. But are they real?

Some scientists confidently say no. All legends about superabilities, psychic phenomena, and other miracles are due to wishful thinking, fairy tales, and superstitions.

They say that our beliefs, enthusiasms, and desires are merely reflections of how brain activity computes our personal world and sense of self. We may enjoy these fantasies, but that doesn't make them real. Nor is there anyone, or even any*thing*, behind this question. That is, what we refer to as "I" or "me" is just a mechanistic illusion that will someday be simulated on a fancy computer. Supernormal powers don't exist.

Maybe that's true.

Maybe not.

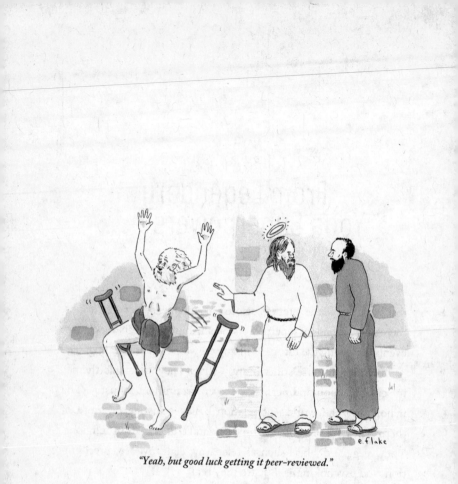

"Yeah, but good luck getting it peer-reviewed."

CHAPTER 1

Introduction

Begin at the beginning and go on till you come to the end; then stop.

—*Lewis Carroll*

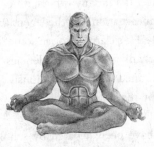

We begin with a simple question: Was Buddha just a nice guy?

Did Buddha's teachings thrive because he was more attractive or charismatic than most, or because he was a great teacher and a tireless advocate of the poor? Or—and here's the core question we'll explore in detail—was it also because he was an enlightened being with profound insights into the nature of Reality, and because he possessed supernormal abilities?

We might ask the same questions about Jesus, Moses, Mohammed, Milarepa, or a host of other historically prominent figures associated with special illumination, wisdom, or grace. Did these people just sport great tans and know how to work a crowd, or did they understand something genuinely deep about the human condition, and our capacities, that is not yet within the purview of science?

If it's too touchy to ask such questions about religious icons, then we may consider a more contemporary figure: The Dalai Lama regularly hosts discussions between scientists and Buddhist monks. Do the Western scientists who compete for a coveted slot at those meetings secretly believe that he's a backward country bumpkin, and they're just humoring him long enough to get their photo taken with a famous Nobel laureate so they can post it on their Facebook page?

Given the glowing praise about those meetings in books and articles authored by no-nonsense science journalists, and a growing list of collaborators hailing from Harvard University, Stanford University, the University of Zürich, the Max Planck Institute for Human Cognitive and Brain Sciences, and many others, it doesn't seem so. But the Dalai Lama takes reincarnation and the legendary yogic superpowers (the siddhis) seriously. He's claimed to see some of them in action, like oracles who accurately divine future tendencies.[6] What does he know that most Western-trained scientists studiously ignore? Could the superpowers actually be real? If so, why haven't we read about them in science magazines?

Such questions have been debated by scholars and by ordinary people for millennia. In modern times, for the most part science has ignored or denigrated the mere possibility of superpowers because such abilities are not easily accommodated by Western scientific assumptions about the capacities of the human mind. It is also sidestepped because any answer offered is guaranteed to seriously annoy someone. If you say yes, "Buddha was just a nice guy," then Buddhists will hurl epithets at you. They may do this in a kind and compassionate way, but you will still have to duck. If you say no, "Buddha was something more," then you will have to dodge objects thrown with equal gusto by both scientists and devotees of other religions. As a result, for the sake of safety the question is usually left unanswered.

There will always be some who are not satisfied with this soft deflection. Cynics feel intense discomfort when questions are raised about the possibility of "something more." They shout accusations of voodoo science, and they form posses to stop what they regard as ominous tides of irrationality from heading our way.[7] Their concerns, bristling on the edge of hysteria, are not without justification. The promise of something secretly powerful, beyond the mundane, has been responsible for untold scams, conspiracies, and witch hunts throughout history. Civilization embraces superstitions and ignores rationality at its peril, so a legitimate case can be made that strenuous protection of hard-won knowledge is necessary.

But here's the rub: It is precisely because civilization must advance beyond superstition that we are obliged to carefully explore our inquiry about the existence of supernormal abilities. The answer is relevant to basic scientific assumptions about the nature of human potential, to the relationships among science, religion, and society, and without hyperbole, to the likelihood that humankind will continue to survive.

In addition, all the nervous fussing one hears about the need to combat superstition, the wringing of hands about looming threats to rationality—such behavior positively drips with emotion, and that presents its own cause for concern. As British psychiatrist Anthony Storr wrote in *Feet of Clay: A Study of Gurus*, "Whether a belief is considered to be a delusion or not depends partly upon the intensity with which it is defended, and partly upon the numbers of people subscribing to it"(p. 199).[8] When it comes to the possibility of superpowers, many are energetically engaged in either strident offenses or frenzied defenses, adding precious little reason to the debate.

But something new can now be brought to the discussion: empirical evidence. Laboratory data amassed over many decades suggest that *some* of what the yogis, mystics, saints, and shamans have claimed is probably right. And that means some of today's scientific assumptions are probably wrong.

If you can't stomach the thought that what you've learned in school might not be completely correct (in spite of the fact that textbooks are regularly revised), then rest assured: This does not mean that all the textbooks must be thrown away. Sizable portions of the existing scientific worldview are quite stable and will remain accurate enough for all practical purposes for a long time.

But it does mean that some of our assumptions, including a few fundamental ideas about who we are and the way the world works, are in need of revision. The newly developing worldview suggests, for example, that it is no longer tenable to imagine that the universe is a mindless clockwork mechanism. Something else seems to be going on, something involving the mind and consciousness in important ways.

After reviewing a substantial body of scientific evidence demonstrating that yoga can significantly improve physical health, *New York Times* journalist William Broad wrote in *The Science of Yoga*:

> While the science of yoga may be demonstrably true—while its findings may be revelatory and may show popular declarations to be false or misleading—the field by nature fails utterly at producing a complete story. Many of yoga's truths surely go beyond the truths of science. Yoga may see further, and its advanced practitioners, for all I know, may frolic in fields of consciousness and spirituality of which science knows nothing. Or maybe it's all delusional nonsense. I have no idea.[9] (p. 222)

Does science really know *nothing* about the more exotic claims of yoga? By the end of this book we'll have discovered that Broad didn't dig deep enough. We actually do know a few things.

Escape to Reality

Many ancient teachings tell us that we have the capacity to gain extraordinary powers through grit or grace. Techniques used to achieve these supernormal abilities, known as *siddhis* in the yoga tradition (from the Sanskrit, meaning "perfection"[2, 5]), include meditation, ecstatic dancing, drumming, praying, chanting, sexual practices, fasting, or ingesting psychedelic plants and mushrooms. In modern times, techniques also include participation in extreme sports, floating in isolation tanks, use of transcranial magnetic or electrical stimulation, listening to binaural-beat audio tones, and neurofeedback.

Most of these techniques are ways of transcending the mundane. Those who yearn to escape from suffering or boredom may dive into a cornucopia of sedatives and narcotics. Others, drawn to the promise of a more meaningful reality, or a healthier mind and body, are attracted to yoga, meditation, or other mind-expanding or mind-body integrating techniques.

Transformative techniques are potent, and like any power they are seductive and rife with pitfalls. Yoga injuries can occur when enthusiasm overcomes common sense.[9] Meditation can lead to extreme introversion, depression, or spiritual hedonism.[10] But the human need to transcend the humdrum is formidable and easily overrides caution. We see this in two of the more popular transformational techniques available today—alcohol and tobacco. These two mind-altering substances are tightly integrated into the economic engines of the modern world. The average household in the United States spends more just on tobacco products and its paraphernalia than on fresh fruit and milk combined, and more on alcohol than on all other nonalcoholic beverages combined.[11]

The World Health Organization estimated that in 2007 the societal cost of alcohol-related diseases, accidents, and violence was over $200 billion a year in the United States alone.[12] The purchase cost of alcohol was even greater, estimated at nearly $400 billion a year in 2008.[13] There is a similar statistic for tobacco.[14] The formidable human desire to escape, just considering these two products alone, costs society trillions of dollars a year. If we included the costs associated with the use and abuse of stimulants and recreational drugs, gambling, and the entertainment industry, the total expense is staggering, a sizable proportion of the world's economy. Humanity seems desperate to escape.

With banks and stock markets on an uncertain roller-coaster ride at the beginning of the twenty-first century, escaping outward has become too risky and too expensive for most people. What about escaping inward? Rarified minds tell us that they have seen something beautiful and glittering in our depths, something that promises a dramatic advancement in human potential. After seriously setting out on that path, most esoteric traditions say that we will eventually encounter genuine extraordinary phenomena, including the acquisition of supernormal powers.[4]

Yoga Superpowers

Classic yoga texts, such as Patanjali's *Yoga Sutras*, written about two thousand years ago, tell us in matter-of-fact terms that if you sit quietly, pay close attention to your mind, and practice this diligently, then you will gain supernormal powers.[15–19] These advanced capacities are not regarded as magical; they're ordinary capacities that everyone possesses. We're just too distracted most of the time to be able to access them reliably.

The sage Patanjali also tells us that these siddhis can be obtained by ingesting certain drugs, through contemplation of sacred symbols, repetition of mantras, ascetic practices, or through a fortuitous birth. In the yogic tradition, powers gained through use of mantras, amulets, or drugs are not regarded with as much respect, or considered to be as permanent, as those earned through dedicated meditative practice.[5]

The promise of these superpowers has little to do with traditional religious faith, divine intervention, or supernatural miracles. As Buddhist scholar Alan Wallace says,

In Buddhism, these are not miracles in the sense of being supernatural events, any more than the discovery and amazing uses of lasers are miraculous—however they may appear to those ignorant of the nature and potentials of light. Such contemplatives claim to have realized the nature and potentials of consciousness far beyond anything known in contemporary science. What may appear supernatural to a scientist or a layperson may seem perfectly natural to an advanced contemplative, much as certain technological advances may appear miraculous to a contemplative.[20] (p. 103)

Yogic wisdom describes many variations of the siddhis. Today we'd associate the elementary siddhis with garden-variety psychic phenomena. They include *telepathy* (mind-to-mind communication); *clairvoyance* (gaining information about distant or hidden objects beyond the reach of the ordinary senses); *precognition* (clairvoyance through time), and *psychokinesis* (direct influence of matter by mind, also known as PK).

For most people, psychic abilities manifest spontaneously and are rarely under conscious control. The experiences tend to be sporadic and fragmentary, and the most dramatic cases occur mainly during periods of extreme motivation. By contrast, the siddhis are said to be highly reliable and under complete conscious control; as such they could be interpreted as exceedingly refined, well-cultivated forms of psychic phenomena.

The more advanced siddhis are said to include invisibility, levitation, invulnerability, and superstrength, abilities often associated with comic book superheroes. All these abilities are also described in one form or another in shamanism and in the mystical teachings of religions. In fact, most cultures throughout history have taken for granted that superpowers are real, albeit rare, and surveys today continue to show that the majority of the world's population still firmly believes in one or more of these capacities.[21]

Mainstream science is not so sure. Many scientists and scholars trained within the Western worldview regard such powers not as supernormal capacities of the human mind, but as superstitions used solely to promote religious faith.[22]

Who's Right?

Who's more likely to be correct about the siddhis—the world's wisdom traditions or today's scientific orthodoxy? We will explore this question not by recitation of amazing stories, or by analysis of religious arguments, or by examination of case reports (although we will look at a few). Rather, we'll concentrate on controlled experimental evidence published in peer-reviewed scientific journals.

We will find that the scientific method is so powerful in discerning fact from fiction that a strong argument can be made in favor of some genuine siddhis. This is an example where scientific evidence trumps previously held assumptions, and it's also a demonstration of the power of science to pull itself up by its bootstraps and to change from within.

This is not to say that this evidence has been warmly embraced. All organized holders of knowledge, whether in scientific or religious contexts, strenuously resist change. We will explore this resistance as well, as it will help us understand why we are only vaguely aware of our true potentials.

What's Ahead

Our approach to this topic is summarized in Figure 1. It shows two basic epistemologies, or ways in which we can know the world—the mystical and the scientific. The mystical includes intuitive and non-rational ways of knowing, such as gut feelings, hunches, visions, and dreams. The scientific involves rational knowing that manifests in three primary forms: (1) empirical, including observation and measurement; (2) theoretical, development of explanatory models; and (3) debate, which includes the skeptical attitude and vigorous deliberations that help maintain the vitality of scientific inquiry.

Figure 1 shows the mystical overlapping science because, like science, mystical experiences have been repeatedly observed, modeled, and debated. Unlike science, mystical experiences have been reported for millennia, far longer than the few centuries of scientific history.

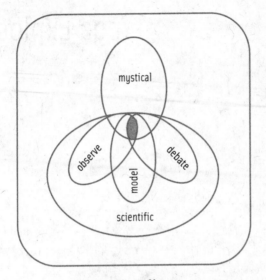

Figure 1. Ways of knowing.

The gray spot in the center of Figure 1 is a place where all methods of knowing overlap. That's the scintillating boundary between the subjective and the objective, the mystical and the scientific. That's where we're headed.

CHAPTER 2

Yoga Explosion

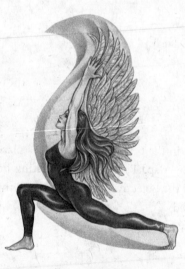

If you look up the word *yoga* on Google's "NGram" search engine, which graphs the appearance of words in millions of books published from 1500 to the present, you will find that it is virtually absent from the English language until about 1900.[23] At that point the curve slowly begins to rise. By 1920 it is clear that *yoga* is becoming more popular, and by about 1960 the usage curve goes exponential. The explosive trend upward shows no signs of slowing, and it graphically reveals that what was once considered a fringe topic within the Western world has become mainstream.

After once-exotic fashions become normal, we forget how long it took for the cultural transitions to take place. Today, for example, Swami Vivekananda is widely regarded as one of the key figures in introducing yoga to the Western world. His speech on Hinduism and interfaith tolerance at the 1893 Parliament of the World's Religions struck an unexpectedly receptive chord.

> "Sisters and Brothers of America," he began, in a sonorous voice tinged with "a delightful slight Irish brogue," according to one listener, attributable to his Trinity College–educated professor in India. "It fills my heart with joy unspeakable . . ." Then something unprecedented happened, presaging the phenomenon decades later that greeted the Beatles. . . . The previously sedate crowd of 4,000-plus attendees rose to their feet and wildly cheered the visiting monk, who, having never before addressed a large gathering, was as shocked as his audience.[24]

Vivekananda was one of the first Western introductions to an Indian guru and yogic scholar. He quickly became a celebrity among prominent authors, scientists, and socialites of the day. But there are always some people who find new ideas strange and uncomfortable, especially the notion of siddhis associated with yogic practice—the "perfections," as they are sometimes called. Consider this scholarly review of Vivekananda's published lectures, which appeared in the *American Journal of Theology* in 1895:

> As our author has given, neither in his book, nor, as far as we are aware, in his life, any evidence that he has yet attained such "perfections," or, indeed, that he has seen any other who possessed them, we simply conclude that he possesses an unlimited assurance, or, in slang phrase, "colossal cheek." . . . We [agree with the] remark that "some of the most important features of

the Hindu's so-called religions are so palpably absurd that the only difficulty in a subsequent age will be to imagine that such things could ever have appeared credible."[25] (p. 405)

Well, here we are in that subsequent age, over a century hence from that review. We can only imagine what the nineteenth-century critic would have thought had he known the changes that were afoot and how Eastern concepts and practices, including yoga and meditation, were about to thoroughly infiltrate Western culture. History has a cruel habit of revealing self-assured pronouncements to be ridiculously shortsighted.

In the 1920s, some elements of the intelligentsia continued to regard yoga practices with a jaundiced eye. A March 3, 1928, news item in *The New Yorker* magazine reflected the sophisticated cosmopolitan view of the day:

> We'd been aware, in a general way, that open-faced house-wives were susceptible to Indian thought, but the ritual came as a big surprise the other evening when, in our persistent search for life's nectar, we joined a group. About two hundred people were sitting on camp chairs. The converts were mostly women—elderly dames with brittle faces and imperfect digestions, the sort of ladies you see on the porch at Lake Mohonk. There were twelve men. Of these, four were colored, four looked like carpet-baggers, and four like William Jennings Bryan. The Yogi wore a long orange robe. (p. 19)

But the barbs were rapidly dissipating. A growing stream of eloquent yogis from India began to establish centers in the West and gain celebrity allies. A key figure in the 1920s was Paramahansa Yogananda, who established the Self Realization Fellowship in Los Angeles and lectured throughout the world through the mid-1930s. In 1946, he published his autobiography, which over the next half century would be read by millions.[26] Just before the turn of the millennium, the publishing company HarperCollins selected his now-classic *Autobiography of a Yogi* as one of the "100 Best Spiritual Books of the [20th] Century."

In the 1930s, Iowa-born Perry Baker, who later changed his name to Pierre Bernard, was instrumental in Americanizing the mystical, soft-spoken yoga of India into the aggressive gymnastics of the cowboy-ethic West. The history of this strange but true tale is recounted in Robert Love's book, *The Great Oom: The Improbable Birth of Yoga in America.*[27] Bernard created today's "yoga-industrial complex," as Love calls it, manifesting as Bernard's two-hundred-acre yoga retreat center on the Hudson River in Nyack, New York. Bernard's enterprise, euphemistically called the Clarkstown Country Club, attracted the pinnacle of society, including academics, politicians, and the wealthy. Initially dismissed as the "Omnipotent Oom" and accused of a rash of nefarious scams and seductions, by the 1930s he had earned fame and fortune, rivaling the celebrity of Charles Lindbergh and appearing regularly in the newspapers' society pages.

About the same time that Bernard was enthralling New Yorkers with his brand of yoga, Jiddu Krishnamurti was rising to prominence. As a young man in India, Krishnamurti had been groomed by Annie Besant and Charles Leadbeater, British founders of the Theosophical Society, to become the spiritual leader of that society. After moving to California, Krishnamurti experienced a mystical awakening and a few years later the unexpected death of his brother. As a result, he became increasingly disenchanted with his role in the Theosophical Society. In 1929, he went out on his own, giving lectures to audiences throughout the world. In 1938, Krishnamurti met Aldous Huxley, a prominent British novelist, whose books *The Perennial Philosophy*, *The Doors of Perception*, and *The Island* were instrumental in popularizing yogic lore, mysticism, and Indian philosophy in the West. Throughout his life, Krishnamurti remained a significant and unique figure in the integration of Eastern thought with Western concerns, ranging from physics to politics. He died in 1986.

In 1955, the US House of Representatives passed a resolution creating the Capitol Meditation Room. "Meditation" at the time was mostly a euphemism for Christian-oriented prayer, but today the distinctions between prayer, meditation, and contemplative practice have considerably blurred. The Capitol Meditation Room was initially supposed to open with the Eighty-Fourth Congress in 1955, but given the studied inefficiencies of politics, it was delayed. The postponement was due to a conflict over an issue of vital importance—the room's decorations. Some members of Congress objected that any form of meditation in the House violated the separation of church and state, so the decorations passed through multiple design revisions before everyone could agree that the room was sufficiently nondenominational.[28]

By the late 1960s, with the psychedelic revolution heating up, the popular press began to track the meditative aspect of yoga, primarily through the popularization of Transcendental Meditation (TM) by Maharishi Mahesh Yogi, and especially by the attention brought to the Maharishi by the Beatles. In 1968, the *Saturday Evening Post* wryly noted:

> The [TM] technique had been lost for many hundreds of years but now had been found again by the Maharishi. . . . The technique, he said, had never been known to fail. Anybody, no matter how skeptical or stupid, could become an adept in the space of four days, during periods of no longer than an hour each day.[29] (p. 24)

Another event in the 1960s that helped to catalyze interest in yoga began when Richard Alpert, a Harvard psychologist and pioneer LSD investigator, traveled to India. While there, Alpert met his guru, Neem Karoli Baba, who gave Alpert the spiritual name Ram Dass. After returning to the United States, Ram Dass wrote *Be Here Now*, one of the first books describing the yogic path, its practices and its philosophy, from a Westerner's point of view. *Be Here Now* (published in 1971) would sell over a million copies and prove to be broadly influential.

In 1970, the secretary of defense, Melvin R. Laird, directed that the Pentagon, like the United States Capitol, should have a nondenominational meditation room.[30] In his dedication speech he said, in part, "Today we are dedicating a room in the Pentagon as a place where the needs of the spirit—the needs of the inner man—can find satisfaction. It is a place where men and women can reflect and pray, and find guidance, as well as inspiration."

After the room was publicized a few years later, it was promptly set on fire and destroyed, possibly on purpose. According to a report in the *Milwaukee Sentinel* newspaper, Pentagon investigators blamed a courier with a history of mental problems who was accused of setting other fires in the building. One hopes that those in charge learned that it wasn't a great idea to allow people with known mental problems to roam freely around the Pentagon.[31] In 1976, a Pentagon Meditation Club was approved by the Office of the Assistant Secretary of Defense.

By the mid-1970s, newspaper stories about yoga and meditation were becoming regular news features, and Lilias Antoinette Moon (better known as Lilias Folan, author of the popular book *Lilias! Yoga and You*) would begin a perennially popular yoga program on PBS television.

In 1973, the *Los Angeles Times* ran a feature article entitled, "Transcendental Meditation: Skeptic Tries It, Comes Away a Believer."[32] Another news item soberly noted that "A 29-year-old yoga instructor found dead in his room in an occult exercise position apparently died of a drug overdose and not, as some followers had suspected, from a dangerous form of meditation"(p. J6).[33] The occult exercise position in question was probably sitting cross-legged on the floor, but the news report didn't provide any details.

By 1977, yoga and meditation centers in metropolitan areas were popping up like mushrooms. Harvey Cox perceptively wrote in his book *Turning East*:

> Why do Americans turn to Oriental religions? The "turn-on" of the 60's and the subsequent turn East were both "a screen of longing for what a consumer culture cannot provide—a community of love and the capacity to experience things intensely." . . .

Several million Americans may indeed have had a brush with Orientalism, but that brush has been relatively superficial if it is based on hatha yoga on television and the first lesson of TM. Even if the neo-Oriental religions have now crested in their popular appeal, they may have left some subtle attitudes which, in the years to come, may resonate and reappear. But it would take a prescient scholar indeed to determine what the form and impact of that reappearance might be.[34]

Cox was right about future trends from the perspective of 1977, but wrong about the cresting of "neo-Oriental" popularity. The crest has yet to wane.

Dangerous Yoga

The Presbyterian Church in the 1970s considered all forms of contemplative practice, including meditation, as "dangerously Roman Catholic," or as "dangerously Buddhist" (p. 61).[35] Three decades later, contemplative practice programs could be found in virtually every Presbyterian seminary in the United States. But not everyone is so progressive. In 1990, the *New York Times* reported:

> Officials in [Toccoa, a small] northeastern Georgia town have canceled a government-sponsored yoga class, bowing to pressure from protesters who contend that yoga invites Devil worship. "The people who signed up for the class are just walking into it like cattle to a slaughter," he said. "Half of yoga is a branch of Eastern mysticism, and it has strong occult influences."[36] (p. 11)

I shudder to think what those protesters thought the other half of yoga was about.

In a more recent expression of this anxiety, the "Lighthouse Trails Research Project," established in 2002, is determined to expose the "dangers of contemplative spirituality." Ironically, it has also assisted in carefully documenting how contemplative practices and meditation have become thoroughly mainstream in evangelical Christian churches. The Lighthouse group is concerned because, in their view, contemplative spirituality is a belief system

> that uses ancient mystical practices to induce altered states of consciousness (the silence) and is rooted in mysticism and the occult but often wrapped in Christian terminology. The premise of contemplative spirituality is pantheistic (God is all) and panentheistic (God is in all). Common terms used for this movement are "spiritual formation," "the silence," "the stillness," "ancient-wisdom," "spiritual disciplines," and many others.[34]

That some are terrified of the concepts of silence, stillness, and ancient wisdom reveals the considerable power of beliefs in shaping our perceptions. Challenges to strongly held beliefs can feel like physical attacks, and they tend to evoke the same types of emotional responses. This is why some fundamentalists argue that the popular Christian-based "Centering Prayer" is unbiblical, or un-Catholic, and perhaps even un-American, because opening one's mind through contemplation and prayer provides an opening for "Satan's influence" (p. 82).[35] Future historians may be surprised to learn that this primeval fear was still very much alive in the twenty-first century.

In October 2010, the Associated Press reported yet another example, entitled "Southern Baptist Leader on Yoga: Not Christianity," but this time even the faithful were saying enough already:

> Louisville, Ky.—A Southern Baptist leader who is calling for Christians to avoid yoga and its spiritual attachments is getting

plenty of pushback from enthusiasts who defend the ancient practice. Southern Baptist Seminary President Albert Mohler says the stretching and meditative discipline derived from Eastern religions is not a Christian pathway to God. Mohler said he objects to "the idea that the body is a vehicle for reaching consciousness with the divine." "That's just not Christianity," Mohler told The Associated Press. . . . Other Christian leaders have said practicing yoga is incompatible with the teachings of Jesus. Pat Robertson has called the chanting and other spiritual components that go along with yoga "really spooky."[37]

Stretching is not Christian? Chanting is really spooky? Despite the good preachers' concerns, as we shall see later, the *practice* of yoga need not have anything to do with religion in any traditional sense, and virtually all religions embrace one or another type of meditation in the form of contemplation or prayer.

Twenty-first-century Yoga

For the segment of the population that is not chronically fixated on medieval fears, yoga and meditation have become enthusiastically mainstream. These ancient practices have been absorbed, transformed, and repackaged into a Western-centric "lifestyle." By 2003, meditation was the cover story in *Time* magazine, and yoga has grown into a multibillion-dollar business with an estimated ten million practitioners in the United States alone. Like sports fans, they eagerly consume classes and products, clothing, themed vacations, videos, books, and magazines. As the *Time* magazine story put it (to prove that they were serious),

Meditation classes today are being filled by mainstream Americans who don't own crystals, don't subscribe to New Age magazines and don't even reside in Los Angeles. For upwardly mobile professionals convinced that their lives are more stressful than those of the cow-milking, soapmaking, butter-churning generations that preceded them, meditation is the smart person's bubble bath.[38]

You know that a trend has firmly entered popular culture when it is targeted by the satirical newsmagazine *The Onion*:

WASHINGTON, DC—According to a Department of Labor report on job retraining, 21 percent of American women are training to be yoga instructors, marking the highest level of female interest in the flexibility-and-spirituality-expansion industry since 1971. "One particular indicator is striking: All but 32 women in New York and San Francisco are now certi-fied yoga instructors, specializing in either hatha, bikram, or ashtanga yoga. . . ."[39]

In 2008, *Yoga Journal*, the premier magazine for yoga aficionados, claimed a reading audience that had ballooned to nearly two million and a paid circulation of 340,000. Other major media outlets have taken notice, as William Broad writes in *The Science of Yoga*:

The *New York Times*, where I work, has run hundreds of articles and in 2010 began a regular column, Stretch. It has profiled ev-erything from studios that offer hot yoga in overheated rooms to a gathering of thousands in Central Park that its organizers called the largest yoga class on record.[9] (p. 2)

Besides the ever-popular Hatha yoga (postures), other yoga forms with different emphases, but sharing the same goal of transcendence, are being explored by growing segments of the Western population, including Bhakti (devotional), Jhana (knowledge), Mantra (words and sounds), Karma (service), Tantra (energy or kundalini), and Ashtanga (also called Raja or royal yoga).

As of June 2012, a Google search on the phrase "yoga studio" returned over five million web pages. Studios can now be found not just in California and New York, but in every US state. Meditation-based programs are paid for by some health insurance companies, and they can be found in prisons, schools, churches, hospitals, airports, industries, the World Bank, the National Academy of Sciences, the *Washington Post*, sports teams including the Chicago Bulls and Los Angeles Lakers, the US Army (Warrior Mind Training[40]), and so on.[41, 42]

Much of the exploding interest is motivated by the scientific confirmation that meditation and yoga, along with dietary changes, provides a huge range of improvements in mental and physical health. Benefits are frequently mentioned in popular media outlets,[35] and that interest is in turn fueled by a steady march of scientific articles. As of February 2012, the National Institutes of Health (NIH) online medical database, known as PubMed.com, listed 2,301 articles with the keyword "meditation." The Institute of Noetic Sciences meditation database, accessible for free through its website, contains citations to over 6,500 articles.

Established benefits of yoga and meditation include improved immune function, lowered blood pressure, treatment and reversal of heart disease, slowed development of prostate cancer, improved focus, memory and concentration,[38, 42, 43] improved quality of life after cancer treatment,[44] positive effects on chronic pain and mood,[45] slower aging, reduced anxiety, reduced infertility, and treatment for otherwise intractable skin diseases.[46] A comprehensive meta-analysis of meditation experiments published in the journal *Psychological Bulletin*, in May 2012, leaves no doubt that meditation differs from mere relaxation and that it significantly benefits a broad range of psychological factors, including emotional regulation, anxiety, relationship issues, attention, and so on.[47]

Those who had been skeptical of meditation but tried it anyway in desperation because of intractable stress or physical injury are often surprised to learn that it is not a religious practice, and being involved in it hardly ever leads to being kidnapped by New Age fanatics. A 2007 article in the *Washington Post* describes such a case:

> Tabitha Benney, a senior program associate at the National Academy of Sciences: "I thought meditation was New Agey and weird, and they would just try to brainwash me and get me to give them all my money. But as soon as I got into that class, and brought my mind and body into the same time zone, I had a sense of wholeness and peace I'd never experienced before. . . ." With the Asian-inspired practices growing in popularity and becoming inexorably less spiritual in nature, workaday schmoes who wouldn't know Vipassana from lasagna now believe we may be able to boost our mental and physical health with brief stress-reduction workouts, much like flattening our abs.[48]

Postural Yoga

Yoga around the world today, including India, is known mostly in the form of postural yoga. These practices typically focus on stretching for flexibility, strength building, balance enhancing, and deep relaxation. Some Hatha yoga studios also include meditation and pranayama (breathing) exercises in their routines.

What is not well known is that this form of yoga is a relatively new invention. Not long ago the idea of yoga focused on postural exercises would have been regarded by leading Indian yogis, including Vivekananda, as primitive at best and repulsive at worst.[49] That's because until recently the only people practicing the stereotyped bodily contortions associated with yoga were street performers, fakirs, and religious ascetics.

The development of postural yoga is a fascinating topic, but to get into the historical details would carry us too far afield from our main focus. It is, however, worth mentioning that yoga as it is known and practiced in the West today, as a quasi-spiritual athletic practice, can be traced not to Patanjali's *Yoga Sutras*, but to an amalgam of traditional yoga poses combined with Swedish gymnastics and British Army calisthenics.[49] In addition, the Western-inspired genius for repackaging traditional wisdom into profit has been so effective that in recent years the Indian government has been busily codifying traditional yogic postures in an attempt to prevent profiteers from patenting or copyrighting what India regards as her time-honored knowledge.

If any one person is responsible for the rise of modern postural yoga, it would be Tirumalai Krishnamacharya, born in South India in 1888. A close second would be his brother-in-law, B. K. S. Iyengar, author of an influential book published in 1966, *Light on Yoga*, and founder of a successful yoga franchise.[9] Krishnamacharya's first female student, a woman born in Latvia in 1899 by the name of Eugenie Peterson, became better known as Indra Devi. From 1947 until 1985, Devi was instrumental in popularizing yoga through books with titles like *Forever Young, Forever Healthy*.[50] She glamorized the practice through her affiliation with movie star devotees, and she became a role model for the benefits of yoga with her vitality (she died in Buenos Aires in 2002 at the ripe old age of 102).[51]

The history of postural yoga is described in detail in Mark Singleton's book *Yoga Body*.[49] He shows how the rise of nationalism in India, ultimately leading to its independence from British rule, was accompanied by a growing interest within India of increasing the power of the body politic by literally strengthening the bodies of Indian citizens. That in turn inspired the metamorphosis of postural yoga from an ancient art practiced by a few to the multinational sport that we know today.

Yoga on the Brain

The Society for Neuroscience, one of the world's largest organizations for professionals involved in brain and nervous system research, publishes a pamphlet called *Neuroscience Core Concepts*.[52] This pamphlet provides a clear statement of what the neurosciences have learned about the mind-brain relationship today. A key finding is that all subjective experiences, all emotional and cognitive processing, and the sense of self are correlated with brain activity. This is usually interpreted to mean that the brain *causes* the mind, but that interpretation is incorrect. What we see are correlations, not causes.

Let's take a short diversion to examine this issue in more detail, because the causation-correlation distinction is important and because it will be relevant to our consideration of the siddhis.

The key point is that correlation does not imply causation. In other words, just because two or more things are closely *related* to each other doesn't mean that one necessarily *causes* the other. As a simple example, flowers turning toward the sun during the day do not cause the sun to move. Or just because forest fires and firefighters tend to be found together doesn't mean that firefighters are causing forest fires. These are trivial examples, but there are many that are more subtle.

This issue is important, because when it comes to understanding the fundamental nature of subjectivity, that is, what a lemon *tastes* like or what a sunset *looks* and *feels* like firsthand, the neurosciences offer no explanation. Some scientists believe that someday, perhaps with vastly improved brain-scanning instruments and new analytical techniques, we'll discover the mechanisms by which the brain literally *causes* subjective experience. They anticipate that we'll be able to build robots with active personal lives or upload our minds to machines so we (or more likely the extremely wealthy) can live forever in shiny metal bodies, or for as long as the batteries hold out.

But so far the promised "mind mechanism" remains utterly mysterious, not just as an engineering problem but also from a core philosophical perspective. How subjective experience can arise from inanimate matter is known as the "hard problem" in the philosophy of mind,[53] and a growing number of scientists are beginning to believe that the effort to find such a mechanism may be a *category mistake*.

A category mistake refers to an error that attempts to combine concepts as though they come from the same category, but actually they don't. For example, asking "What is the square root of 16?" is a perfectly good question because a square root is a process that acts upon numbers, and 16 is a number. But asking "What is the square root of an apple?" isn't a well-formed question because it attempts to mix different categories. Likewise, asking what are the neural mechanisms that *cause* subjective experience might be a category mistake because the question assumes that *objective* and *subjective* belong to the same category. If they don't, then the search for physical mechanisms cannot succeed.

As the philosophical hard problem continues to tantalize neuroscientists, it is interesting to note that some neural correlates have been found for some mystical and spiritual experiences.[54] This implies that reports of those states are probably not fabricated. They are real in the same sense that our perceptions of reality are closely correlated with brain activity, so people having spiritual experiences aren't just making them up. But what we can't know with today's technology is whether such reports are merely illusions or hallucinations.

From a psychiatric perspective, those who report profound religious experiences, such as the sensation of transcending the physical world, may be diagnosed as suffering from a brain disorder called "hyperreligiosity,"[55] an obsessive interest in religious concepts. Damage to certain areas of the brain, such as the posterior parietal cortex, can indeed inhibit one's sense of being located "here" and "now," and that can in turn lead to certain types of behavior that are assumed to be symptoms of an underlying disease, rather than to something "real."

This assumption is not without merit. People who have a lesion in the posterior parietal cortex do tend to believe in miracles and ESP more than the average person with an intact brain, and they tend to agree with the following statement:

> I often feel so connected to the people around me that I feel like there is no separation; I feel so connected to nature that everything feels like one single organism; and I get lost in the moment and detached from time.[56]

Does this mean that advanced yogis and meditators—the poster children for enthusiastic endorsers of transcendent experiences—also have misfiring posterior parietal cortexes?[56] Not necessarily. Some brain activity is engaged in processing information, but a good deal is also engaged in *inhibiting* the processing of information. If this were not so, we'd quickly become overwhelmed with sensory input, which some have estimated to be a trillion times more information than we can consciously experience.[57]

So if something goes haywire in an area of the brain that was actively inhibiting our ability to sense that separation is an illusion, then wouldn't we expect that person to become very interested in mysticism? After all, he or she is now experiencing reality as "oneness," whereas before the brain was actively blocking those perceptions. Alternatively, if after twenty years of meditation we find that a yogi's posterior parietal cortex begins to inhibit certain perceptual blocks, then wouldn't we expect him to start experiencing the oneness of the universal Self, or the ancient Hindu adage that Atman equals Brahman?

Changing Perspectives

While these questions simmer, science marches on, and old assumptions about the brain-mind relationship continue to evolve. This is reflected in popular books such as Sharon Begley's *Train Your Mind, Change Your Brain*.[58] The paradigm shift is quickening because it is now scientifically acceptable—thanks largely to the Dalai Lama's cachet—to study contemplative practices. Through this multicultural line of research, scientists are finding that the brain-mind relationship is much more intimately connected than previously imagined, and the brain itself is far more malleable.

It is worth remembering that not long ago the idea of a malleable brain/mind was considered ridiculous. As Begley explained, "Just a few years before, neuroscientists would not even have been part of this conversation, for textbooks, science courses, and cutting-edge research papers all hewed to the same line, as they had for almost as long as there had been a science of the brain" (p. 5).[58]

The next revolutionary shift will occur when other assumptions about the brain-mind relationship are put to the test. A Georgetown University professor of East Asian and Buddhist studies, Francisca Cho, forecasts where the current trend is headed:

> Buddhism has taught for twenty-five hundred years that the mind is an independent force that can be harnessed by will and attention to bring about physical change. "The discovery that thinking something effects just as doing something does is a fascinating consonance with Buddhism," says Francisca Cho. "Buddhism challenges the traditional belief in an external, objective reality. Instead, it teaches that our reality is created by our own projections; it is thinking that creates the external world beyond us. The neuroscience findings harmonize with this Buddhist teaching."[58] (pp. 13–14)

In its most radical form, this line of thought is perfectly compatible with claims about the supernormal powers of the yogic siddhis. Yogic teachings and practically every other tradition based on thousands of years of introspection have learned from firsthand experience that the mind is not reducible to the brain. From those traditions it's the other way around—brain activity reflects a subtler version of mind than the neurosciences have yet imagined.

Does this mean that present assumptions adopted by the neurosciences are vanishing, including the assumption that supernormal siddhis are impossible? No, not yet. There are still major clashes between assumptions and beliefs that continue to constrain the discussion. As Sharon Begley noted in the conversations between scientists and the Dalai Lama,

> Mind "enjoys a status separate from the material world," argues the Dalai Lama. "From the Buddhist perspective, the mental realm cannot be reduced to the world of matter, though it may depend upon that world to function." As far as the scientists were concerned, however, the proposition that the mind is some ethereal, incorporeal, even spooky entity that can act back on the brain to alter its physical or chemical structure is at best quaint.[58] (p. 153)

> As adamantly as they reject dualism, scientists are nevertheless beginning to appreciate the causal power of purely internal mental processes to give rise to a biological effect. That intrigued the Buddhists, with [physicist and Buddhist scholar] Alan Wallace suggesting that the discovery of the power of thought to alter the brain . . . "calls for scientific research into these different strata of consciousness that does not just assume they're all dependent upon the brain." "From the scientific perspective," said [neuroscientist] Richie Davidson, "the honest answer is that we don't know" how mental processes influence the physical brain. "The same is true from the Buddhist perspective," [Buddhist monk] Jinpa said to laughter.[58] (p. 156)

In spite of the good-natured laughter, the orthodoxy is not ready to take *all* the claims of advanced meditation seriously. The siddhis are still too spooky to contemplate. But there is progress.

Deity Yoga

Certain meditative practices of Buddhist monks involve creating and maintaining sequences of exceptionally detailed visual imagery. Advanced meditators report that these vivid images can be held for minutes to hours, and indeed the practice requires this because the images are so complex. Neuroscientists regarded such a claim to be absurd. Their understanding of the brain convinced them that it was virtually impossible to hold mental imagery for more than a few seconds.

It took the Dalai Lama to goad the neuroscientists into conducting a test to see who was right—the meditators or the scientists. Maria Kozhevnikov of George Mason University and her colleagues took up the challenge by testing experienced monks at Sechen Monastery in Kathmandu.[59] She used two standard tests of visual memory, one involving rotation of mental images and the other holding complex images in memory.

The monks used two types of meditation. *Deity Yoga* involves generating and holding a three-dimensional color image of a deity surrounded by his or her divine entourage. The other type of meditation is called *Open Presence*, in which attention is broadly distributed without focusing on any experiences, images, or thoughts that may arise. The claim tested about Deity Yoga was the assertion that highly complex images could be mentally maintained for minutes to hours. Kozhevnikov also tested nonmeditators and meditators who did not engage in their practice prior to the test.

The results showed that all the groups performed at the same level before meditation, but after meditation, the Deity Yoga practitioners, according to Kozhevnikov, "demonstrated a dramatic increase in performance on imagery tasks compared with the other groups. Therefore, [Deity Yoga] specifically trains one's capacity to access heightened visuospatial memory resources via meditation, rather than generally improving long-lasting imagery abilities" (p. 645).[59]

That sounds like an unassuming success until we read the rest of the article, in which Kozhevnikov reports that "we are not certain how long this state of access to heightened visuospatial resources might last. . . . During the informal interviews, some of the practitioners reported that the powerful state of identification with the deity can be sustained for several hours or more, whereas others reported that the effect lasted for only approximately 20 to 25 [minutes]" (p. 645).[59]

To emphasize, she reported *minutes to hours*, as compared to seconds, which was what neuroscientists had previously believed was the limit. In addition, the description of a "dramatic increase" in visual memory does not adequately highlight just how much the monks' imagery ability shifted from before to after meditation. For the Open Presence and control participants, there was no statistical difference in the ability to hold imagery. But for the Deity Yoga participants, the difference was associated with odds against chance ranging from a million to a billion to one.

Odds Against Chance

We must now take a semitechnical detour. In this book I often express results of experiments in terms of "odds against chance," so it's important to understand what that phrase means. Experiments involving human performance are usually interested in comparing how people perform in two or more conditions. For example, to test if performing Deity Yoga really does improve mental imagery, we could compare people's performance on a visual memory task before and after they practiced that form of yoga. The "null hypothesis" is the conservative expectation that there is *no difference* in performance.

So now we go ahead and conduct the experiment, and then we perform a statistical comparison on the resulting data. Statisticians use probabilities called "*p* values" (*p* meaning probability) to indicate how unlikely the outcome of an experiment would be if chance alone were responsible for the results. Say the results of our experiment were strong enough that the effect we measured would only occur 1 in 20 times when no effect was present (i.e., it was a pure chance outcome). In that case we'd say that the associated p value was 1/20 or $p = 0.05$. We could also say that the *odds against chance* for the experiment were the inverse of 1/20, or 20 to 1. Throughout this book, I cast p values into odds because more people are used to casino terms like "odds" than abstract terms like "p values."

Now say that we've run an experiment and it produced odds against chance of a million to one. This means that if we conducted this same experiment a million times, *and* the effect we observed was just due to dumb luck, then we would see results as good as what we actually observed only one in a million times. The result might still be due to chance, but it would be one heck of a lucky day.

With this amazing outcome, we are presented with two possible interpretations: either (1) we were extremely lucky or (2) our guess that there should be no difference in performance (as noted earlier, we called this the "null hypothesis") might be wrong.

In either case, we now have a good reason to believe that the difference we observed in the experiment was *probably* not due to chance. This is referred to in technical jargon with a confusing double negative: "rejection of the null hypothesis." To determine exactly *what* caused the difference we observed requires much more research, but at the initial stage when we just want to know if there are any differences at all, this outcome provides ample motivation to keep on investigating. In particular, even if an experiment produces extremely high odds against chance, this doesn't mean that the effect we're interested in is *proven*.

All the annoying cautions and qualifications commonly used in scientific lingo—it *might* be this, it *could possibly* be that, the *purported* results *may perhaps* be such and such—sound like a curious lack of enthusiasm, or an unwillingness to take a firm stand. But the prudence is intentional. It prevents existing knowledge from coagulating into unshakable dogma, which is the forte of religious faith.

Also, just because a statistical test ends up with huge odds against chance doesn't necessarily mean that the effect we were measuring is what we imagined it to be. To gain that sort of confidence it takes many independent scientists repeatedly examining the same effect in different ways, and for the results to be consistent on average. As we'll see, this is indeed the case for experimental tests of certain supernormal siddhis.

One other thing: I should clarify what I mean by the word *experiment*. Flipping a coin to see if you get heads or tails could be called an experiment in the sense that it's a slightly more attentive version of an ordinary experience. It also doesn't cost much in terms of time, effort, or money. By contrast, in later chapters the evidence I will be referring to involves collections of dozens to hundreds of experiments. Each of those experiments may have involved several scientists, and a typical study can easily take one or two years to complete. Collectively, these studies have involved thousands of person-years to conduct, document, and publish in peer-reviewed scientific journals.

I mention the effort involved in scientific experiments because oftentimes when research studies are reported in the popular press, years of effort are compressed into a few paragraphs, so it's easy to gain the impression that research is quick, cheap, and easy. That is rarely the case.

Summary

Yoga in the West was once considered an exotic Eastern import. Today it's a core component of a burgeoning sports industry, one with a special niche as a quasi-spiritual form of exercise. The health benefits of postural or Hatha yoga, which is available in many forms, are now widely accepted, but it is not generally known that the methods taught in yoga studios today were derived both from ancient yoga asanas (postures) and from Western-style gymnastics and calisthenics. The benefits of the meditative side of yoga are also increasingly well accepted, but meditation as a means of consciousness transformation, especially the ancient relationship between meditation and superpowers, is still considered a taboo topic and is avoided in polite conversation. The next two chapters explore why this is so.

CHAPTER 3

Other Realities

In the history of the collective as in the history of the individual, everything depends on the development of consciousness.

—*Carl Jung*

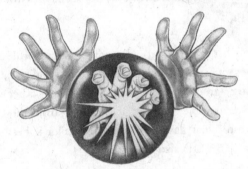

Most metaphysical, occult, and esoteric schools believe in another, deeper, hidden reality beyond the mundane world.[60] The mystics, saints, and geniuses who blazed trails in those transcendental realms have given us many marvelous stories, and their insights are the foundations of most of our religions. Of course, similar tales are told by the delusional and the insane, and this muddies how those experiences should be interpreted. The line between genius and madness is notoriously thin.[61, 62]

When scholars of religion began to compare these "other reality" experiences across cultures—from overwhelming feelings of cosmic oneness to a sense of intense meaning underlying mundane physical appearances—they noticed some intriguing similarities. What the mystics described appeared to be a repeatable human experience, suggesting that beneath variations in appearance something very real was going on. Perhaps the most famous synthesis of this idea, called "perennialism" by scholars, was expressed by Aldous Huxley in his 1944 book *The Perennial Philosophy*. Huxley described this as

> the metaphysic that recognizes a divine Reality substantial to the world of things and lives and minds; the psychology that finds in the soul something similar to, or even identical with, divine Reality; the ethic that places man's final end in the knowledge of the immanent and transcendent Ground of all being.[51] (p. 95)

Why is it that mystics across the millennia, regardless of their religious beliefs, cultural background, or educational training, seem to provide better agreement on the nature of that "other world" than most scientists are able to agree on anything from the causes of climate change to what flavor of ice cream flavor is best? The British philosopher Alan Watts also noted this

> . . . single philosophical consensus of universal extent. It has been held by [men and women] who report the same insights and teach the same essential doctrine whether living today or six thousand years ago, whether from New Mexico in the Far West or from Japan in the Far East.[63] (p. 168)

Psychiatrist and psychedelic researcher Rick Strassman, similarly struck by the strong subjective agreement about nonordinary realities, proposed the following:

Foolish, arbitrary thinking can hardly reach this degree of consensus. Not without sarcasm, Ken Wilber said: "Eighty-three hallucinating schizophrenics couldn't organize a trip to the bathroom, let alone Japanese Zen."[63] (p. 2964)

It is worth noting that not all scholars of mysticism embrace perennialism. Some are instead "constructivists"; they see clear differences among esoteric traditions and practices, and they argue that those differences lead to entirely different states of consciousness and experience. Still others accept that because mysticism is grounded in human experience, and humans haven't changed much in the last ten thousand years (or more), some form of perennialism is probably valid, but nevertheless culture still strongly shapes how we *interpret* our experiences.

Beyond the fine points of how to properly interpret esoteric experiences, many mystical traditions also claim that there are methods one can use to develop a direct realization of these states. According to psychiatrist and meditation researcher Roger Walsh:

> Comparison across traditions suggests that there are seven practices that are widely regarded as central and essential for effective transpersonal development. These seven are an ethical lifestyle, redirecting motivation, transforming emotions, training attention, refining awareness, fostering wisdom, and practicing service to others. Contemplative traditions posit that meditation is crucial to this developmental process because it facilitates several of these processes.[64] (p. 28)

Modern physics has achieved its own version of the perennial philosophy through the development of quantum theory. While many workaday physicists shudder over popular misinterpretations of their precious mathematical models, the founders of quantum mechanics were keenly aware of the radical philosophical changes brought about by their new theory. They wrote about it extensively, and most of them ended up sounding like full-blown mystics. For example, we find in the writings of the Nobel laureate physicist Erwin Schrödinger: "I have . . . no hesitation in declaring quite bluntly that the acceptance of a really existing material world, as the explanation of the fact that we all find in the end that we are empirically in the same environment, is mystical and metaphysical" (p. 94).[65]

Like classical physics, which provides mathematical models of the world, quantum theory also provides accurate descriptions of how the physical world operates. In both cases the mathematics are not actually about the world itself but are symbolic approximations. However, a big difference between classical and quantum theories is that the former physicists imagined that they were describing the actual world itself; that is, they thought that their equations and reality shared a one-to-one correspondence. With that knowledge, physicists gained enormous confidence in understanding how the world works by simply manipulating mathematical equations.

That confidence is what led the Greek mathematician Archimedes to proclaim, "Give me a lever long enough and a fulcrum on which to place it, and I shall move the world." This symbolic approach to understanding the world is at times astonishingly accurate, which is why physics has gained such high prestige among scientific disciplines.

But with the introduction of quantum theory, physicists found themselves forced to acknowledge that their models were now describing *descriptions* of the world, rather than the world itself. This was literally a shift from physics to metaphysics. Many, including Einstein, rejected this change. As integral philosopher Ken Wilber put it:

Both the old and the new physics were dealing with shadow-symbols, but the new physics *was forced to be aware of that fact*—forced to be aware that it was dealing with shadows and illusions, not reality. Thus, in perhaps the most famous and oft-quoted passage of any of these theorists, Eddington eloquently states: "In the world of physics we watch a shadow-graph performance of familiar life. The shadow of my elbow rests on the shadow table as the shadow ink flows over the shadow paper. . . . The frank realization that physical science is concerned with a world of shadows is one of the most significant of recent advances. . . ."

To put it in a nutshell: according to this view, physics deals with shadows; to go beyond shadows is to go beyond physics; to go beyond physics is to head toward the meta-physical or mystical—and that is why so many of our pioneering physicists were mystics.[66]

Shamanism

Perhaps the oldest tradition associated with the deliberate evocation of mystical experience is shamanism, an ancient animistic belief that assumes everything is alive and that certain people (shamans) are able to interact with living spirits. Forms of shamanism have been traced back through the mists of Stone Age prehistory. It can be found in every indigenous culture, and shamanism is still vibrantly alive today not only in less developed countries, but also at the leading edges of the contemporary world. It is possible to purchase shamanic drumming apps for the iPhone, and Google finds a million websites containing the word *shamanism*.

The anthropologist Weston La Barre emphasized the ancient importance of shamanism by noting that the typical interpretation of "the world's oldest profession" was not prostitution, but shamanism. The shaman was an essential part of every tribe—the first doctor, priest, oracle, and keeper of wisdom, all embodied in the same person.[67] The shaman's profession required him, or her, to reliably enter visionary states on demand. The use of psychedelic drugs was brought to a high art for this purpose, possibly including the *Amanita muscaria* mushroom, which some believe was the basis of the transformative beverage called Soma by early Brahmin priests. Soma may have been the catalyst for the ancient revealed Hindu texts, the Vedas, and ultimately yoga as a transformative practice.[68] Other methods developed by shamans included music, dancing, controlled breathing, drumming, fasting, breathing intoxicating vapors, and meditation.[69]

Why did shamanism arise in virtually all ancient cultures? Harsh environments and ever-present dangers faced by the earliest humans undoubtedly led them to adopt anything or anyone that helped the tribe survive and thrive. This was the special gift of the shaman, but shamans didn't have a free ride. If their visionary assistance proved to be faulty, either their own tribe or another would probably eliminate them. Over centuries of trial and error we can imagine that the techniques for reliably entering visionary states, developed and passed down by generations of shamans, would have become progressively more effective.

Shamanism was wildly popular thousands of years ago, but why are people still walking around today with shamanism apps on their smartphones? Why is there a renaissance among scholars who are revisiting ancient shamanistic practices,[70] and why does the general public take shamanic journeying workshops and ecotourism field trips to distant lands to experience *ayahuasca*, *ibogaine*, and other traditional hallucinogenic plant medicines?

One reason is that it is now possible for anyone to gain access to the world's once-secret indigenous teachings, over the Internet, in a flash. While spiritual and shamanic *stories* do not provide the raw experiences that many are interested in, they do capture the lore. And the lore is saturated with the possibility of gaining mind-blowing, transformative experiences of other realities.

Psychedelics

Another reason for the resurgence of shamanism, proposed by psychiatrist Roger Walsh, is a consequence of the 1960s psychedelic revolution. As Walsh puts it, the widespread use of psychedelics in the '60s unleashed experiences of such intensity and impact that they shook the very foundations of society. Suddenly millions of people found themselves blasted into types of experiences and states of consciousness that were, quite literally, beyond their wildest dreams. A Pandora's box of heavens and hells, highs and lows, trivia and transcendence poured into minds and societies utterly unprepared for any of them. For perhaps the first time in 2,000 years since the Greek Eleusinian mysteries, a significant proportion of a Western culture experienced powerful alternate states of consciousness.[64] (p. 4)

Millions of people, thrust into visionary states that challenge traditional ways of life, are a threat to any government, which is undoubtedly why almost all the psychedelic plants that grow naturally throughout the world have been criminalized or subjected to preposterous public relations campaigns to "just say no." Say no to the revelation of a whole new reality? As Daniel Pinchbeck wrote in his book *Breaking Open the Head*:

> In the sophisticated contemporary world, it seems absurd to propose that the dismissed and disgraced psychedelic compounds might be real doorways to neighboring dimensions, and within those other realms there are beings we can contact who are waiting to welcome us with disconcerting glee. It is even more absurd to suggest that some of those beings resemble our folkloric archetypes, because they are the source for those archetypes in the first place.[71] (p. 206)

But the fact remains that practically anyone who explored those realms has returned stunned after learning that the shamans, and the yogis, were probably right: Everyday reality is just one provincial way of perceiving the world. There are others that are equally valid, and it's in some of those worlds where the supernormal resides.

Those who have not experienced these states may assume that all visionary experiences, including those resembling the yogic siddhis, are hallucinatory. In some cases this is undoubtedly true, especially when powerful mind-altering substances are abused by teenagers looking for kicks. But serious students of shamanic practices universally acknowledge that some supernormal phenomena are accessed in these states. As psychedelic evangelist Terence McKenna once said, "Shamans speak of 'spirit' the way a quantum physicist might speak of 'charm'; it is a technical gloss for a very complicated concept" (p. 155).[71]

Trips and Tryptamine

The US government's panicky reaction to the psychedelic revolution of the 1960s resulted in a screeching halt to all scientific research on these compounds. A half century later, the hysteria has begun to settle down and research is under way again. One drug being studied is a powerful psychedelic that is endogenous to the human body: DMT (*N,N*-dimethyltryptamine).[63] In Rick Strassman's book *Inner Paths to Outer Space*, he describes a typical experience induced by DMT:

> Time no longer passes in its normal manner, but instead seems suspended or subsumed in an eternity containing past, present, and future. Space is no longer limited, but at the same time, all existence rests in the smallest possible unit of space. The self can now hold and feel at utter peace with life, good and evil are seen in their deepest reality, and the nature of free will is clearly perceived.
>
> . . . It is known as a certainty that there exists an unimaginably powerful creator and sustainer of reality, and of you in particular. This creator is unborn, uncreated, undying, and unchanging. The ecstasy and searing bliss accompanying such experiences, though previously unequaled in intensity, is nev-

ertheless less striking than the peace and equanimity that supports and underlies this bliss.[63] (p. 1162)

This description is virtually identical to the yogi's ecstatic state of deep absorption, called *samadhi*. Strassman was aware of this, so he proposed that endogenous DMT may be activated in advanced meditation, and that this may be the biochemical cause, or at least a correlate of, mystical experiences. Because of the striking similarities in how these states are described, one could even predict that DMT-induced and meditation-induced ecstasies might share similar reports of transpersonal connections, including clairvoyance and telepathy as described in the *Yoga Sutras*. And they do.

Strassman, like many Western-trained scientists, found it difficult to imagine that the mystical experiences described by the participants in his studies were "real" in any ontological sense. The repeated similarities of those experiences, and the insistence that these were not hallucinations, eventually forced him to reconsider. He wrote:

[The] presence of DMT may suggest a previously unappreciated fluidity, permeability, or plasticity of the membrane separating us and other worlds. This barrier, then, may exist more inside of us than outside of us—in inner rather than outer space. Therefore, travel across great distances in outer space may not be the only way to reach worlds that are different from our own, seemingly remote in time and space. Moreover, it may be unnecessary to restrict this search using methods based upon a view of reality limited to what is physical and measurable.[63] (p. 1505)

A sign that something truly astonishing can happen in these states was reported by another modern psychedelics researcher, neuroscientist Roland Griffiths of Johns Hopkins University School of Medicine. Like Strassman, Griffiths was interested in the frequent reports of mystical experiences induced by psychedelics. In 2008, he and his colleagues reported a remarkable finding on long-term behavioral changes as a result of taking psilocybin—a compound synthesized from mushrooms—under carefully controlled conditions.[72]

Griffiths's team tested thirty-six adults who were not experienced users of hallucinogenic drugs, but who did have some type of regular participation in religious or spiritual activities. Fourteen months after their use of psilocybin in the laboratory, over half of the participants rated the psilocybin-induced experience as being among the five most personally meaningful experiences of their entire lives.

That finding was consistent with an earlier follow-up study of seven seminary students who had received psilocybin in the context of a religious service some twenty-five years before. These lasting transformative experiences demonstrate how powerful psychedelics can be (both positive and negative), and it lends credibility to the yogis' description of the life-transforming nature of meditation-induced enlightenment experiences.

Extreme Sports

Another approach to transcendence in the modern age is extreme sports. In ancient times putting oneself at risk for adventure wasn't sport—it was called daily life, or catching dinner. But today climbing mountains, white-water rafting, surfing the big waves . . . these are a siren call for both the hardy and the foolish. One of the draws is the ecstatic feelings that can accompany conquering the impossible. Another is the lure of transcendence.

Maria Coffey explored the connections between extreme sports and transcendence in her book *Explorers of the Infinite*. The book's subtitle says it all: *The Secret Spiritual Lives of Extreme Athletes, and What They Reveal About Near-Death Experiences, Psychic Communication, and Touching the Beyond*. In story after story, Coffey recounted how adventurers who pushed themselves to the limit experienced the whole panoply of mystical and psychic phenomena. After recounting a harrowing tale, the athlete telling his or her story would often add in hushed tones: "I have no doubt that it was real. . . . I was not hallucinating and I'm not crazy" (p. 211).[73]

Summary

The aboriginal otherworldliness of shamanism, the bizarreness of psychedelic trips, and the transcendent experiences of extreme sports (including Tantric sexual practices) are some of the reasons why stories about these topics are enthusiastically embraced by the public. What fan of sex, drugs, and rock and roll doesn't already believe that there's a little transcendental magic in that explosive mix? But when the exciting tales of other realities touched through these practices, or supernormal powers evoked by them, are soberly presented as *real*, the only sounds heard in the sedate halls of academia are the echoes of footsteps scurrying away.

CHAPTER 4

Mysticism and Miracles

A miracle does not happen in contradiction to nature, but in contradiction to that which is known to us of nature.

—*Saint Augustine*

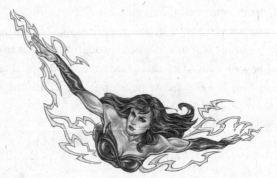

Because we're exploring the supernormal, it is useful to spend a bit of time pondering miracles. The word *miracle* comes from the Latin *miraculum*, or "object of wonder." It refers to an extraordinary event presumed to be caused by something beyond all known natural or earthly forces. As such, miracles are attributed to super*natural* or divine causes. By contrast, a *marvelous* event is regarded as an unusual but perfectly normal event that's not yet understood. If a marvelous episode is really spectacular, it might be called super*normal*. The siddhis are thus marvelous, and not miracles.

Both miracles and marvels are characterized by a sense of awe and with what Walter Huston Clark called "a descent into madness, described as the *mysterium tremendum*, or the mystery that makes one tremble. . . . In these cases the sense of wonder is tinged with a religious intimation of overwhelming significance" (p. 773).[74]

In the sophisticated, postmodern, twittering twenty-first century, miracles are regarded by nonreligious Westerners as quaint beliefs of bygone days. Many scientists and scholars regard them as arcane superstitions that, as described by Islamic scholar Zia Inayat-Khan, are "intrinsically obfuscatory and incompatible with rational thought."[75]

And yet, when the Pew Forum on Religion and Public Life asked thirty-five thousand Americans in 2007, "Do you believe in miracles?,"[76] a whopping 79 percent responded yes. Among those with religious affiliations 83 percent said yes, which is not especially surprising, but even among the religiously unaffiliated more than half—55 percent—also said yes.

This tremendous faith in the miraculous—manifestations of the divine—gives incorrigible skeptics indigestion, but it is clear that the idea of miracles provides something important that people need to believe in, and that neither an aseptic science nor a sneering atheism can override. Cynics are quick to explain this need as due to a puerile lack of control in the face of health or financial crises, or to a lack of education. But those explanations are too facile. Healthy minds crave meaning and purpose as much as the body craves food, maybe more. Miracles provide a sense of purpose, of something "bigger" than oneself, something worth living for.

Purported miracles are so powerfully attractive that traditional religious authorities are quick to constrain rumors whenever they occur. Whether it's the face of Jesus appearing on a grilled cheese sandwich, a bleeding statue of Mother Mary, or something more profound—like the miracle of Fatima, Portugal, in 1917, where thousands of witnesses, including skeptics, were stunned to see something unearthly in the sky[77]—miracle control squads investigate and package official stories, which are then marketed to the faithful with the proper spin.

The Catholic Church is especially adept at public relations efforts when it comes to miracles, because to maintain central authority church leaders found it necessary to prevent the masses from withdrawing their faith from existing authorities and redirecting it toward miraculous interlopers. It would not do to have people worshipping a grilled cheese sandwich, although stranger things have happened. Consider the many miracles associated, for example, with the Catholic ritual of the Eucharist.[78]

Miracle stories also persist within the modern materialistic worldview because, as David Weddle writes in *Miracles: Wonder and Meaning in World Religions*, they "challenge established views of what is possible and impossible, and in so doing shatter the modern illusion that scientific constructions of reality are absolute" (p. 123).[79] In other words, miracles let us enjoy our technological gadgets and scientific marvels, but they also provide room for the intuitive sense that the real mysteries of the universe, those nagging existential questions about meaning and purpose, have yet to be touched upon by science. Until that happens in a serious way, miracles will remain an ever-popular fascination.

So are miracles merely wishful thinking, or are some of them real? Do genuinely extraordinary events occur that are currently beyond the capacity of science to explain?

Some will argue that this is not a suitable topic for science to address. Surely miracles are at the wrong end of the rationalism scale, so why not let the professors of religious studies and the philosophers debate this and leave science out of the fight? The answer is easy—it's not just scientists who won't touch this taboo. Scholars won't go there either. According to Rice University historian of religion Jeffrey Kripal:

> Whereas such marvels are vociferously denied (or simply ignored) in the halls of academic respectability, they are enthusiastically embraced in contemporary fiction, film, and fantasy. We are obviously fascinated by such things and will pay billions of dollars for their special display, and yet we will not talk about them, not at least in any serious and sustained profes-

sional way. Popular culture is our mysticism. The public realm is our esoteric realm. The paranormal is our secret in plain sight. Weird.[80] (p. 6)

Weirder still is that the academic discipline that is founded on and fueled by tales of the mystical, the miraculous, and the paranormal—the study of religion—is just as stubbornly defiant as science is when it comes to investigating these events. Kripal writes:

The study of religion as a discipline, as a structure of thought, *as a field of possibility*, has severely limited itself precisely to the extent that it has followed Western culture on this particular point, that is, to the extent that the discipline constantly encounters robust paranormal phenomena in its data—the stuff is *everywhere*—and then refuses to talk about such things in any truly serious and sustained way. The paranormal is our secret in plain sight too.[80] (p. 7)

Because of this entrenched cultural stubbornness, I believe that science is actually obligated to investigate miracles as neutrally and as thoroughly as it possibly can. The only alternative are those dismal debunking exercises, which are tolerable when there are high-quality reasons to suspect bunk. But charging recklessly into miracles while shouting, "I'm a debunker!" guarantees that if something genuine is going on, it will quietly slink away.

There is another reason to be tolerant of the mystical and miraculous, expressed by the most celebrated rationalist of the twentieth century, Albert Einstein. He wrote:

I maintain that cosmic religious feeling is the strongest and noblest incitement to scientific research. Only those who realize the immense efforts and, above all, the devotion which pioneer work in theoretical science demands, can grasp the strength of the emotion out of which alone such work, remote as it is from the immediate realities of life, can issue.

Those whose acquaintance with scientific research is derived chiefly from its practical results easily develop a completely false notion of the mentality of the men who, surrounded by a sceptical world, have shown the way to those like-minded with themselves, scattered through the earth and the centuries. . . . A contemporary has said, not unjustly, that in this materialistic age of ours the serious scientific workers are the only profoundly religious people.[81] (pp. 21–22)

Einstein maintained that mystical realizations are not just brain malfunctions, at least not when experienced by true genius. They are instead an essential means of leaping beyond the rational and accessing what intellect alone cannot grasp.

If it is indeed the case that there are ways of knowing that transcend the rational, and our geniuses are telling us that it is precisely this that sparks genuine breakthroughs, then avoiding this mystery is akin to societal suicide. Einstein's "religious feeling," which he carefully stripped from its faith-based connotation, may well be the only way to pull ourselves up by our bootstraps into new realms of knowledge.

Theocrats were not pleased with Einstein's and others' heretical claim that no church authority was necessary to have or to interpret these experiences. Catholic priest Tony Anatrella, speaking about the "world of youth today," expressed concern when he wrote:

There are currents of philosophy and wisdom without God that have come from Asia and the East that are interesting as such, but they are not religions, and they are being put forward and distorted at the present time. Nevertheless, they do not represent a large movement. With this mentality, you have to be "cool," "zen" and quiet, that is, feel nothing and be in a muffled torpor.[82]

From Father Anatrella's perspective, the Catholic Church apparently equates contemplative practice with something like getting buzzed on wine or stoned on marijuana. This is a serious misunderstanding because meditation is about expanding and clarifying awareness, not about contracting it.

Mysticism Defined

What is the religious feeling that Einstein admired? The father of American psychology, William James, provided one of the clearest definitions. It involves four key characteristics: The first is *ineffability*, meaning it cannot be adequately expressed in words; it must be experienced to be fully understood. As James wrote in his classic book *The Varieties of Religious Experience*, "No one can make clear to another who has never had a certain feeling, in what the quality or worth of it consists" (p. 371).[83]

The second characteristic is a *noetic* quality, meaning that the mystical experience is felt to be a state of knowledge. According to James, noetic refers to "states of insight into depths of truth unplumbed by the discursive intellect. They are illuminations, revelations, full of significance and importance, all inarticulate though they remain; and as a rule they carry with them a curious sense of authority for after-time" (p. 371).

The third feature is *transiency*, referring to the time course of these experiences. In objective time, spontaneous mystical experiences may last only a few moments, or in rare cases a few hours. Subjectively they seem to last far longer.

The fourth is *passivity*, in which the onset of the mystical state might be sparked by meditation or other means, but once that state begins it is no longer felt to be under control by the mystic. According to James: "[It is] as if [the mystic] were grasped and held by a superior power" (p. 372).

Interpreting Mysticism

Religious scholars have long debated the nature of mystical experiences. Are they hallucinations, or do they reflect a veridical picture of Reality *as such*, as the mystics universally claim? As this debate evolved, two primary definitions of mystical experience have been proposed, known as *constructivism* and *essentialism*. The constructivist approach assumes that mystical events have been part of human experience ever since there were humans, and in particular they were happening to people long before the establishment of formal religions. But the way that the raw experience manifests, how it is interpreted, and how it becomes embedded into religious doctrines is strongly shaped by culture, language, and beliefs.[84]

By contrast, the essentialist interpretation assumes that mystical experiences transcend local cultural and religious beliefs, and that there are common phenomenological characteristics among these experiences that can be found throughout history and across all cultures.[85]

The connection between the mystical and the miraculous in the context of this book is that yoga is a path for practical mystical development, and that path *explicitly includes* the development of miraculous phenomena, or more precisely, of supermarvelous phenomena that *appear* to be miraculous. Walking on water, manipulating matter with the mind, and foreseeing the future are all said to be produced through gaining expertise in mystical states.

As yoga has become progressively more Westernized to make it palatable to the Western mind, its mystical and miraculous connotations have been sanitized. The supernormal marvels of the siddhis have been reframed into the amazing wonders of lower stress and better health without drugs.[51] This is understandable because while the majority of the population privately expresses belief in miracles, only certain, limited kinds of miracles that do not directly challenge religious beliefs can be discussed in public. Also, the concept that it is possible to transform good ol' Bubba Six-Pack into miracle-worker Baba Sixaji through diligent yoga practice exceeds most people's boggle threshold, even though it may well be true.

Marvelous Stories

In Buddhism, the existence of advanced powers is readily acknowledged, and it is clear from the *Tipitaka*, or Pali Canon, the doctrinal texts of Theravada Buddhism, that Buddha expected his disciples to be able to attain these abilities, but also to not become distracted by them.[79] A professor of Buddhist and Tibetan Studies at the University of Michigan, Donald Lopez Jr., describes that Buddha was

> believed to possess all manner of supernormal powers, including full knowledge of each of his own past lives and those of other beings, the ability to know others' thoughts, the ability to create doubles of himself, the ability to rise into the air and simultaneously shoot fire and water from his body. . . . He was believed to have passed into nirvāna at the age of eighty-one, although he could have lived "for an aeon or until the end of the aeon" if only he had been asked to do so.[86] (p. 8)

In the Pali Canon, Buddha describes other "supranormal" powers as follows:

> When a monk has thus developed and pursued the four bases of power, he experiences manifold supranormal powers. Having been one he becomes many; having been many he becomes one. He appears. He vanishes. He goes unimpeded through walls, ramparts, and mountains as if through space. He dives in and out of the earth as if it were water. He walks on water without sinking as if it were dry land. Sitting crosslegged

he flies through the air like a winged bird. With his hand he touches and strokes even the sun and moon, so mighty and powerful. He exercises influence with his body even as far as the Brahma worlds.[87]

Because the Buddhist tradition accepts supernormal powers, but science does not, the Mind and Life Dialogues between the Dalai Lama and scientists have been fruitful and engaging as long as the topic of the supernormal is not broached. The Dalai Lama has gainfully and repeatedly tried to raise this topic in his discussions, but to little avail. For example, in the second Mind and Life conference in 1989, he was engaged in a discussion with Harvard psychiatrist Allan Hobson when the following exchange took place:[88]

DALAI LAMA: There are instances where small children recollect their past life very vividly.

ALLAN HOBSON: But what is the evidence that they have recollected correctly and accurately? There must be solid, quantitative, documentary evidence, not simply testimony.

The Dalai Lama then described a case involving a girl from India who recalled names of people she claims she had known in previous lives. You can imagine the scientists present at this exchange struggling to contain their eye rolling. Philosopher Patricia Churchland and neuroscientist Antonio Damasio proposed that the girl might have heard stories from others. The Dalai Lama patiently explained that ordinary explanations were considered and they do not seem to explain this case. Churchland and Damasio then wondered if this is real, then why wasn't it more common?

The scientists discussing this topic can be forgiven for not being familiar with the relevant evidence; no one can be an expert in everything. But had they looked at the National Institutes of Health

Pubmed.com online bibliography, and searched for the word *reincarnation*, they would have found a number of interesting articles. One is by University of Virginia psychiatrist Jim Tucker, who in 2008 published a review of cases suggestive of reincarnation.[89]

Worldwide over twenty-five hundred such cases have been studied in detail, most often in locations where reincarnation is culturally accepted, including India, Sri Lanka, Turkey, Lebanon, Thailand, and Burma. Similar cases have been found on every continent except Antarctica. Tucker's article began by acknowledging that this research was not well known, but that the work begun in the 1960s by University of Virginia psychiatrist Ian Stevenson has been taken seriously by skeptics who have studied the evidence. Tucker writes:

> The *Journal of the American Medical Association* reviewed one of [Stevenson's] books in 1975 and stated that "in regard to reincarnation he has painstakingly and unemotionally collected a detailed series of cases . . . in which the evidence is difficult to explain on any other grounds." In addition, Carl Sagan, the late astronomer, was very skeptical of nonmainstream work but wrote, "There are three claims in the [parapsychology] field which, in my opinion, deserve serious study," with the third being "that young children sometimes report details of a previous life, which upon checking turn out to be accurate and which they could not have known about in any other way than reincarnation."[89] (p. 244)

Tucker then describes a typical reincarnation case:

> The average age when subjects begin reporting a past life is 35 months. Some make their statements with detachment, but many show strong emotional involvement in their claims. Some cry and beg to be taken to what they say is their previous family. Others show intense anger, particularly toward killers

in cases in which the previous personality was murdered. In general, the stronger the evidence for a connection to the previous life, the more emotion the child shows when talking about that life.

. . . The subjects usually stop making their past-life statements by the age of six to seven, and most seem to lose the purported memories. This is the age when children start school and begin having more experiences in the current life, as well as when they tend to lose their early childhood memories.[89] (p. 245)

Tucker continued with an example of an American case, a child named Sam Taylor, who, one day when he was a year and a half old,

looked up as his father was changing his diaper and said, "When I was your age, I used to change your diapers." He began talking more about having been his grandfather. He eventually told details of his grandfather's life that his parents felt certain he could not have learned through normal means, such as the fact that his grandfather's sister had been murdered and that his grandmother had used a food processor to make milkshakes for his grandfather every day at the end of his life.[89] (p. 246)

Many conventional explanations for these cases have been debated. So far the conclusion, according to Tucker, is that "the processes that would be involved in such a transfer of consciousness are completely unknown, and they await further elucidation" (p. 247).[89]

Note that none of these cases involves hypnotic "past-life regressions," or any other form of guided suggestion. There are too many confounds in such cases to make that sort of evidence useful for assessing whether the memories are veridical. For this reason, in Stevenson's and now in Tucker's research, only cases involving very young children have been studied where there is good reason to believe that the children are not faking it.

Returning to the Mind and Life conference, in his conversation with Hobson, the Dalai Lama raised the issue of knowledge obtained in dreams:[88]

> DALAI LAMA: I know some Tibetans who lived in Tibet prior to the 1959 uprising. Before their escape from Tibet, they did not know about the natural trails and passes by which to get over the Himalayas into India. Some of these people I met had very clear dreams of these tracks and, years later, when they actually had to follow the actual trails, they found that they were already familiar with them because of the very clear dreams they had had previously.

> ALLAN HOBSON: This is a so-called precognitive dream and there are many examples of this in the West as well. I would like to defer discussion of that until later, as it is an important question. (p. 59)

A while later, the Dalai Lama returned to other phenomena that are taken for granted by the Tibetans:

> DALAI LAMA: There are certain people who feel they have out-of-body experiences while dreaming.

> ALLAN HOBSON: This has not been studied in the laboratory, but it is easy to imagine how such a state could arise since it is possible to hallucinate practically anything during dreaming. (p. 63)

The Dalai Lama continued to press the issue:

> DALAI LAMA: There are accounts of people experiencing this sense of leaving their body, actually perceiving things in the external

world, and later being able to recall events that presumably took place there, even to the point of being able to read a book in someone else's house. Has there been no scientific investigation of this type of testimony?

ALLAN HOBSON: That is correct, there has been no scientific investigation of these. But I would like to discuss this issue because I think that the issue of precognitive dreams, out-of-body experiences, and claims of previous lives, all have a problem in common for science. . . . The question is: How can we advance any of these claims above the status of what we would call testimony and anecdote? (p. 64)

This exchange highlights a central problem in dealing with discussions of miracles. Scientists meeting with the Dalai Lama are undoubtedly interested in anything he has to say, but having been selected as scientific or scholarly experts in their fields, they probably feel a certain pressure to behave like experts, even when they don't know what they're talking about. The discussion panel's answer to the Dalai Lama's questions about reincarnation, precognition, and veridical out-of-body experiences might have been a more modest "I don't know." Instead, they asserted that science has not studied these issues, or they gave the impression that the reason there is no scientific evidence is because the beliefs are not true. In fact, there is substantial evidence, and the results confirm that at least *some* of the Tibetans' beliefs are almost certainly true.

Medical Miracles

Reluctance to accept anything that smacks of miracles is not just the case in science. It is also common in medicine. Physician Rex Gardner studied a number of miraculous healings described by the Venerable Bede, an English monk in the Middle Ages who was renowned for his scholarship. Bede is well regarded as an accurate historian, and yet his written works also include accounts of medical miracles. Gardner was challenged by this anomaly, and so he looked into contemporary cases of medical miracles and published his findings in the *British Medical Journal* in 1983. He began by acknowledging the following:

> The modern scholar is above believing in miracles, in fact from his view point "scholarship" and "belief in miracles" are mutually exclusive terms. . . . So far as I have been able to discover, no Bedan scholar in recent times has asked that simple question which seems the obvious one to us in medicine. Were these patients healed as described or not? Secondly, is it a useful search? Can miracles ever be proved?[90] (pp. 1927–28)

Gardner reviewed seven cases; I'll briefly describe two.

CASE 1: In 1977, an eleven-month-old boy with signs of a lung disease that is nearly always fatal was treated without success. He was taken to a healing service by a Pentecostal pastor, and five days later he was markedly better. At a follow-up physical four years later he was completely normal.

CASE 2: In 1975, a student physician suddenly became ill and was admitted to the hospital. Four physicians diagnosed her with Waterhouse-Friderichsen syndrome, a bacterial blood infection that leads to massive internal bleeding. No one had ever recovered from that particular diagnosis in that hospital. Later that evening, four separate groups prayed for her recovery, and in the same evening there was a sudden improvement in her condition. She subsequently recovered completely. On her admittance to the hospital her chest X-rays showed extensive left-side pneumonia and a completely collapsed middle lobe of the lung. Forty-eight hours later, the X-ray showed a perfectly clear chest. In addition, in the acute phase of her illness her left eye had developed intraocular bleeding, which left her completely blind in that eye. She eventually regained full vision.

Gardner concluded:

A number of case histories of "miraculous" healings in the past 30 years have been presented in which independent corroboration is possible. It is noteworthy that in most cases members of the British medical profession still in practice were actively taking part. No attempt has been made to prove that miracles have occurred, such proof being probably impossible. . . . These cases have been paired with miracle stories recorded by Bede and his contemporaries, which up to now have not been considered historically admissible. They have normally been discarded as mere copies of New Testament incidents, or of prototype lives such as that of St Antony produced to add stature to a local saint. . . .

It is my contention that we can now treat their writings with even greater respect than has up to now been possible. They, and the saints whose lives they portray, prove to be men of greater stature than we have hitherto believed. . . . The simplest explanation appears to be that, being no longer expected or even welcome, miracles no longer occurred.[90] (p. 1932)

Is the same true of the supernormal siddhis? As we will see, most of the elementary siddhis can be found in ordinary people today, including those with no yoga or meditation practice. But what about the more dramatic superabilities, such as levitation or invisibility? Are these also dependent on cultural acceptance, expectation, or belief? Perhaps so, but fortunately when it comes to occasional medical miracles, they still occur in ordinary people for unknown reasons.

In 1993, Brendan O'Regan and Caryle Hirshberg of the Institute of Noetic Sciences surveyed the medical literature to see if remarkable cases like those described by Rex Gardner and others were still being reported.[91] They were surprised to find in the medical literature 1,385 documented case studies of "spontaneous remissions," the medical euphemism for unexpected, startlingly sudden, and complete healings.

Of those cases, 1,051 referred to spontaneous remission of cancer and 334 to other diseases. These were all instances where patients were diagnosed with X-rays, biopsies, and so on, and they either refused treatment, no treatment was available, or they were treated by methods that were available but were known to be insufficient for a cure. And all the patients fully recovered.

The orthodox medical response to such spontaneous cures is that the original diagnoses were mistaken. In some cases that critique may be correct, and it is also true that spontaneous cures are rare compared to those that are not cured. But they do happen.

Beyond Yoga

Tales of supernormal mental powers are not unique to the yogic tradition. Most of the same abilities are described in Catholicism as *charisms* and in Islam as *karāmāts*.[92] In Judaism, *nahash* or divination may be practiced by a *zaddik*.[93, 94] In Tibetan Buddhism, the term is *ngön she*, meaning heightened awareness. These same abilities are described in detail in the eminent Buddhist text *The Flower Ornament Scripture: The Avatamsaka Sutra*.[95] All shamanistic traditions are saturated with such tales.

An important distinction between the yogic view of the siddhis, as compared to the religious, is that yoga presents a practical path for developing these abilities whereas most religions assume that these abilities are divinely inspired, meaning they are God-anointed gifts rather than extraordinary human skills.

Indeed, those who display the siddhis within religious contexts are often considered blessed with the divine or cursed by the demonic. This ambivalence presents a problem for how religious authorities respond to reports of supernormal events, because the interpretation becomes as much of a political act as one of moral discernment. Witnessing a supernormal event can be powerfully seductive, and that presents a threat to traditional authority. Why should one lend devotion or allegiance to a church that promises miracles some day in the future, or preaches about miracles of the past, when a saintly person is performing miracles right here, right now? By contrast, yoga takes a more pragmatic approach to displays of the siddhis because they are not considered divine, nor are they as tightly wound into the power struggles that seem to be endemic in all human affairs, including organized religions.

The Catholic charisms are among the better-known supernormal abilities in Western culture. They include the familiar, such as *clairvoyance* and *precognition*, exemplified by the prophecies of Saint Gertrude, Saint Hildegard, Saint Birgitta of Sweden, Saint Catherine of Siena, and Saint Teresa; *supernormal healing*, as told in copious stories of miracle cures; and *dominion over nature and creatures*, such as the remarkable case of Saint Alphonsus Liguori, who, when ordered by a major general of the Redemptorists to eat a plate of veal, refused and instead converted it—so the story goes—by the holy sign into a delicious cod cutlet.[96]

Then there is *levitation*, of which there are between two hundred and three hundred historical cases in the descriptions of the saints, including Saint Joseph of Cupertino (1603–1663). Saint Joseph was observed to levitate by thousands of witnesses, usually in broad daylight, over a period of thirty-five years. Reports can be found in witnesses' private diaries and in depositions provided under oath, including 150 eyewitness reports from popes, kings, and princesses.[97] Purely secular cases of levitation also exist, including most famously that of the Scottish medium Daniel Dunglas Home (1833–1886).[98] Like Saint Joseph, Home was observed to levitate in daylight by dozens of prominent witnesses. Not a single case of fraud was ever discovered.

Other charisms include *bilocation*, in which the mystic is observed to appear in two distant places at the same time; *fragrances*, or the "odor of sanctity," issuing from the mystic's body or clothes; *inedia*, or complete abstinence from food or drink for long periods of time, without harm; *infused knowledge*, or the supernormal ability to gain wisdom without studying; *incorruption*, the absence of the normal decay of the body after death; *discernment of spirits*, which in the Catholic context means interacting and knowing the difference between angels and demons; and *luminous irradiance*, a glowing light surrounding the heads, faces, and sometimes the whole bodies of mystics.

Finally, we have a charism with a distinctly Catholic spin that sounds like a Johnny Cash tune: *incendium amoris*, or the "burning fire of love." As described by Montague Summers,

> Saint Maria Maddalena de Pazzi, who was transformed by sudden overwhelmings of love, "for her face, losing in a moment the extreme pallor which had been produced by her severe penances and her austere cloistral life, became glowing, beaming with delight, and full; her eyes shone like twin stars, and she exclaimed aloud, crying out "O love! O Divine Love! O God of Love!" Moreover, such was the excess and abundance of this celestial flame which consumed her, that "in the midst of winter she could not bear woolen garments, because of that fire of love which burned in her bosom, but perforce she cut through and loosened her habit." She was even compelled to run to a well and not only to drink a quantity of icy cold water, but to bathe her hands and her breast, if haply she might assuage the flame.[96] (p. 71)

Skeptics

One interpretation of the superpower similarities described across all religions is that they are reflections of the same, genuine siddhis. Another interpretation is proposed by party poopers who are determined to reframe these reports in reductionist scientific terms. Psychologist James Leuba, who wrote about and proposed a strictly reductionist psychology of religion and mysticism in the early part of the twentieth century, described yoga as a "connecting link between the religious intoxication of the savage and the mysticism of the higher religions" (p. 46).[99] His withering critique of Patanjali's description of yoga asserted that the lofty goal of achieving the state of oneness associated with samadhi, and the siddhis associated with that state, were

> obviously nonsense. The Yogin cannot substantiate his claim to a knowledge of the thoughts of other persons, of the time of his death, or of his present and future incarnations; concentration upon the moon does not give him an intuitive knowledge of "the arrangement of the stars." A careful reading of Yoga discloses, however, that magical omniscience and omnipotence are not taken too seriously. After all, the Yogin keeps his eyes first of all on deliverance from pain. That, in truth, is the gross purpose of Yoga.
>
> We know in any case that he is much deceived in the magical powers he ascribes to himself. His self-deception, the corresponding self-deception of the user of drugs, and, as we shall see, of the classical Christian mystics, constitute one of the most pathetic chapters of human history. To aim so high and to fall so low is in truth both deep tragedy and high comedy. The stupefied Yogin is one of the blundering heroes and martyrs that mark the slow progress of humanity.[99] (p. 46)

Perhaps I'm misunderstanding Leuba's remarks, but I get the sense that he did not approve of Patanjali's tales of the siddhis.

Summary

The awe and the emotional power underlying most religions are fueled by tales of the supernormal and the supernatural. Even in the age of science, belief in a wide range of marvels and miracles remains widespread. Some of those beliefs can be traced to disenchantment with the materialistic, purposeless worldview that science has advanced over the past few centuries. Other beliefs are reinforced by the attraction of more comforting religious stories. But beyond belief, similarities in supernormal abilities and mystical experiences reported throughout history and across cultures suggest that something genuinely remarkable may be going on. Others strenuously disagree and argue that all talk of marvels and miracles is nonsense. Skepticism in response to the unexpected is healthy; excessive doubt may be less beneficial. Let's see why.

CHAPTER 5
Unbelievable

As soon as I touched the broad, empty bowl, it became heaped with hot butter-fried luchis [flatbread], curry, and rare sweetmeats. I helped myself, observing that the vessel was ever-filled. At the end of my meal I looked around for water. My guru pointed to the bowl before me. Lo! the food had vanished; in its place was water, clear as from a mountain stream. . . . The sage picked up from a near-by table a graceful vase whose handle was blazing with diamonds. "Our great guru created this palace by solidifying myriads of free cosmic rays," he [said].[26]

—Paramahansa Yogananda, *Autobiography of a Yogi*

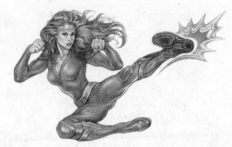

Seriously? Blazing diamonds and solidified cosmic rays?

I remember when I first read this passage as a teenager. I was filled with wonder and delight. Unlike fairy tales, which I enjoyed and knew to be fantasy-embellished parables, this was presented as a factual autobiography—the real stuff. I envied Yogananda for having witnessed such marvels.

Years later, after earning advanced degrees in electrical engineering and psychology, I was working on various projects at AT&T's Bell Laboratories. At the time, Bell Labs was one of the world's premier scientific organizations, famous for inventing some of the stalwarts of modern technology, from the transistor to the laser and the cell phone. Like most of my colleagues at Bell Labs, after decades of education in engineering and science I learned that when one encounters stories of "real" miracles, the first thing that's supposed to come to mind is not awe or wonder, but exasperation at how anyone beyond the age of five could possibly believe in such nonsense.

I was taught that breathless tales of mind over matter or extrasensory perception—when presented as literally true—were at best magical thinking and at worst an impending psychiatric problem. The scientific culture taught me that Swami Yogananda would have benefited more, not from a bowl filled with imaginary butter-fried flatbreads, but from a fine selection of antipsychotic medications.

But I was also troubled by a nagging sense that something important was missing from my university courses, something real that mythology and fairy tales were pointing to as metaphors. I later discovered to my surprise, and relief, that the same sense of loss was an unspoken secret among many of my colleagues at Bell Labs. I eventually found to my amazement that this was true also within the larger scientific world. Despite official amusement, dismissal, and scorn aimed at stories like Yogananda's, I found that quiet interest in advanced human potentials, including psychic and mystical experiences, permeated the mainstream. And not just the industrial research mainstream, but also the academic, scientific, government, medical, and military mainstreams. In such contexts you quickly learn not to talk about such things too openly, because a few people will invariably turn red, become loudly upset, and cause trouble. So these interests percolate underground.

Quietly. Persistently.

This odd state of affairs makes it possible in the Western world to advance from preschool through postdoctoral positions and never learn about—or in many cases even hear about—serious scientific investigations of psychic or mystical experiences.

By investigations I don't mean what's portrayed on the proliferation of reality TV shows about ghostbusting or other forms of paranormal entertainment. What you see on the oxymoron of "reality TV" is a virtual drama crafted for one reason only—to grab and hold your attention. Real ghost hunting involves endless hours waiting in strange places for something unexpected to happen. On those rare occasions when something does go bump in the night, there is no way to know with certainty if the bump was an anomalous glitch in your perception, a faulty instrument reading, or a potentially meaningful piece of data.

What I mean by investigations are laboratory studies using gold-standard scientific methods, with results published in peer-reviewed professional journals. It's that line of research that you don't often hear about. Instead, what you learn in school is predicated on the belief that mechanistic materialism—the prevailing scientific dogma—is sufficient to explain *everything* in the natural world. This is what the vast majority of college science textbooks teach, implicitly or explicitly.

This dogma is accepted because for many practical concerns it works. It has led to real advances in knowledge. It allowed us to advance from the Dark Ages to the moon and beyond. But it also leads to a worldview that seems to exclude the possibility of genuine siddhis. I would emphasize "seems" because in fact this is not actually true when the modern understanding of the physical world is considered, as we shall see.

And realistically it's not a trivial problem to find individuals who can repeatedly demonstrate supernormal abilities on demand within the constraints of strict laboratory controls. I believe that such people probably do exist, but those with the most talent studiously avoid the limelight, and for good reason. When the occasional superstar emerges from obscurity and provides a public demonstration, the media frenzy surrounding such events quickly devolves into a circus atmosphere where separating truth from fiction becomes impossible. A few millennia ago there were no twenty-four-hour news or "infotainment" television channels, but the ancient sages were already familiar with the problem of media circuses, and they had much to say about the use of siddhis for entertainment or egotistical reasons. We'll discuss that later.

Don't Look Here

The clash between private and public beliefs sustains a powerful taboo that ensures that scientific interest in the supernormal continues to simmer below the surface. The taboo is reinforced by self-appointed vigilantes who feel compelled to police an unwritten social commandment not to speak of certain topics, at least not in serious tones. An example is a television program called *Bullshit!*, which aired on the Showtime premium cable channel from 2003 to 2010. This program was a vehicle for vigorously attacking anyone or anything that the hosts, two stage magicians, regarded as nonsense. That included psychic ability. The program's provocative title came about because

> the series would contain more obscenity and profanity than one would expect in a series dealing with scientific and critical inquiry, but [it was] explained that this was a legal tactic because, "if one calls people liars and quacks one can be sued . . . but 'assholes' is pretty safe."[100]

While some objects of that program's invective may have deserved harsh treatment, no scientist is willing to risk becoming the target of public ridicule, or to ask for trouble by quarreling with lawyers who crafted a clever way to finesse the libel laws.

The reinforced stigma also translates into a statistic that highlights the stunning power of this taboo. In spite of the fact that opinion surveys consistently show that a majority of the world's population is fascinated with psychic phenomena, fewer than 1 percent of the world's accredited universities have even a single faculty member known for his or her scientific interest in these phenomena.[101]

What's wrong with this picture? Billions of people are spellbound by the supernormal, yet the topic is flatly ignored by over 99 percent of the institutions of higher learning worldwide. The entertainment industry zealously responds to public interest with its perennial rash of programs with supernormal themes,[102] so we might expect some mainstream universities to also capitalize on that interest. After all, universities are always looking for ways to attract more students, which is one reason why it's possible to earn doctorate degrees focusing on, say, "The semiotics of *Star Trek*" or "The archetypal hermeneutics of *Buffy the Vampire Slayer*."

While scholarly works on *Star Trek* or *Buffy* might sound frivolous to a scientist's ears, they actually touch upon an important perspective. As Rice University scholar of comparative religions Jeffrey Kripal notes in his book *Mutants and Mystics: Science Fiction, Superhero Comics, and the Paranormal*, our ideas about the possible are far more inhibited and reserved than we might like to think. The humanities specialize in seeing through the surface of our stories, including the story of science, which rests upon multiple layers of assumptions. As these layers are progressively penetrated, the rock-solid worldview created by science begins to dissolve, and it eventually leads to a fascinating realization. As Kripal puts it, through "intimate, often invisible influences in language, culture, and religion [human beings] are being constructed—*they are being written*" (p. 28).[103] We will revisit this concept, which is relevant to our theme on science and the siddhis, in the last chapter of this book.

Outside of Kripal's works, the fact remains that it is almost forbidden in the orthodox academic world to even entertain the possibility that some of the siddhis, or any supernormal or paranormal abilities, might be real. There are very few exceptions to this rule. Supernormal abilities are instantly conflated with supernatural beliefs, and no serious (Western-trained) scholar believes in the supernatural anymore, right? It's embarrassing to think that anyone ever did.

There is also a cultural bias at play. This becomes more apparent when we look at how unusual mental experiences are regarded outside the Western world. In India, cases of multiple personality disorder are diagnosed among a tiny fraction of psychiatric patients, a mere 0.015 percent.[104] In the United States, the figure is hundreds of times greater, a whopping 10 percent.[105] This difference may arise because the Western mind is more prone to fracturing than the Eastern mind, due to cultural expectations. That is, the ideal Western ego is an isolated, ruggedly independent, separate entity, all alone in a dead universe devoid of meaning or consciousness—the leather-faced cowboy, pondering empty thoughts.

Social psychologists have found that buying into that gloomy worldview leads to a reduction in beneficial behavior such as helpfulness and empathy.[106] By contrast, advanced meditators, many of whom have reported psychic and mystical experiences, display significantly increased capacities for compassion and vastly improved physical and emotional well-being.[107]

What We Are Taught

British astrophysicist Sir Arthur Stanley Eddington once wrote, "It would be a shock to come across a university where it was the practice of the students to recite adherence to Newton's laws of motion, to Maxwell's equations and to the electromagnetic theory of light."[108] Nobel laureate physicist Brian Josephson adds to this that "it is equally a shock, today, to find reputable scientists categorically asserting, in the manner of dogma, the impossibility of phenomena such as extrasensory perception."[109] But such assertions nevertheless do occur, and regularly. It is instructive to explore why this is so, because this is one source of the persistent taboo we are discussing and the reason that science and scholars have so fervently resisted looking at the supernormal.

Other than in Eastern philosophy and religious studies courses, most Western college students are unlikely to take any classes that mention the word *siddhi*. It is possible to find an occasional psychology course on weird beliefs that refer to psychic or mystical phenomena, but most of those are within the context of learning what people who lived in premodern times believed, or what people on the edge of schizophrenia believe today, rather than whether their stories could possibly be true.

Other courses, offered from psychological or neuroscience perspectives, are designed to pound into students the idea that such topics are dangerous pseudosciences, and thus heartily deserving of mockery and shame.[110] These so-called critical thinking courses are designed to reinforce a kind of scientistic catechism. Students who survive such classes learn to accept that any positive evidence they may encounter for "miraculous" abilities is definitively explained away as delusions, scams, or signs of psychosis. Those who disagree, because such explanations do not jibe with their own experience, learn to remain quiet.

I once gave a lecture for a university's "Psi Chi" group, the international honor society for student psychologists. I presented the results of experiments my team had conducted investigating how one person's focused thoughts aimed at another person, isolated at a distance, affected the remote person's autonomic nervous system. We found that this version of the "feeling of being stared at" phenomenon demonstrated under strictly controlled conditions that sometimes those sensations were quite real.[111]

The students listened attentively and asked good questions afterward. Then as the meeting was adjourning, a red-faced faculty adviser sitting in the back of the room suddenly jumped up, rushed to the front of the room waving a batch of papers, and hurriedly passed them out to the students. Curious about this strange behavior and the adviser's flushed appearance, I borrowed one of the papers and saw that it contained a long list of books and articles written by hard-core debunkers. The adviser breathlessly explained to the students that this was his list of recommended reading about the paranormal, and that he expected them to read it. What he didn't say was that this was his attempt to eradicate any possible "contaminating" influence I might have had.

The students learned from their adviser's spectacle that they were expected to disavow any interest in the supernormal. They timidly followed that demand and I never heard from any of them again. I wish I could say that this episode was an exception to the rule, but unfortunately it isn't.

What Our Textbooks Say

In many introductory psychology courses, professors hope to dissuade their students from believing in miracles or "the paranormal" by telling them that believers are more dogmatic than skeptics, or that they lack critical thinking skills, make more errors on reasoning, come from a lower socioeconomic status, have lower intelligence, have parents with lower educational levels, score higher on psychoticism scales, score lower on social conformity, and are more depressed, dissociated, and hyperactive.[112–115]

Professors will sometimes admit that most of the studies resulting in such disparaging outcomes were conducted by incurable skeptics, or that the results are much weaker and ambivalent than usually portrayed.[116] But somehow those caveats aren't mentioned. Then they recommend that teachers of psychology inform themselves about these issues by

> reading journals like the *Skeptical Inquirer* and books like Hansel's . . . critique of parapsychological research, and secondly, by teaching courses about the paranormal. . . . Until skeptical

psychologists take such teaching seriously, students and the general public will continue to rely for information about the paranormal on sources such as the *Readers' Digest,* the *National Enquirer,* and Steven Spielberg films.[112] (p. 214)

Other professors exclusively assign readings from skeptical books that lump together topics like "ghosts, voodoo, the UFO conspiracy, and other paranormal phenomena" into a single pot, or they smugly purport to explain "why people believe in weird things." Such books provide naive explanations for these phenomena using "principles of valid science."[117]

I hope that students understand that the holier-than-thou debunking exercises in skeptics' magazines, and the outrageous tales in tabloids and awe-inspiring films, are not the sort of credible information one needs to make informed decisions about complicated topics. Books that exclusively focus on explaining away weird beliefs may help readers feel intellectually superior to their "uneducated" brethren, but when those readers rehash the entertainment they've just read and turn them into college textbooks, we're headed for trouble.

A case in point is a popular introductory psychology textbook by Keith Stanovich, entitled *How to Think Straight About Psychology.* In it, Stanovich states that the reason scientists have become impatient with ESP research is because "the area is tainted by fraud, charlatanism, and media exploitation" (p. 25).[118] The implication is that scientific investigations of psychic phenomena are uniformly blemished and therefore lack credibility. This would be a powerful argument if it were true. It isn't.

The truth is that in the entire history of laboratory investigations of these phenomena, spanning more than a century, there is one case of proven fraud and two or three suspected cases. Compared to the number of cases of scientific misconduct in conventional disciplines, ranging from outright data fabrication to duplicate publication and plagiarism, this domain is positively saintly.[119] Of course, fraudulent mediums were popular in the late-nineteenth and early-twentieth centuries, and today there continue to be scam artists who pose as psychics. But *rampant* fraud or media exploitation among *scientific* studies of psychic phenomena? Pure fiction.

Stanovich then blithely explains why academic psychologists no longer pay any attention to ESP:

> The reason that ESP, for example, is not considered a viable topic in contemporary psychology is simply that its investigation has not proved fruitful. Therefore, very few psychologists are interested in it. It is important here to emphasize the word contemporary, because the topic of ESP was of greater interest to psychologists some years ago, before the current bulk of negative evidence had accumulated. . . . The results of the many studies that have appeared in legitimate psychological journals have been overwhelmingly negative. After more than 90 years of study, there still does not exist one example of an ESP phenomenon that is replicable under controlled conditions.[118] (p. 187)

Variations of the above assertions can be found in many college psychology textbooks, and it paints a sober reason to ignore psychic research. But the plain fact is that there is no body of "overwhelmingly negative" results. As we'll see, reviews of several classes of psychic (or *psi* for short) phenomena have been published in peer-reviewed professional journals, and they show overwhelmingly *positive* results.

Anecdotal Claims

I've encountered many other fictions claimed about the evidence for psi. In 2000, I was a member of a panel discussion on ESP for a Public Broadcasting Service television show called *Closer to Truth*. One of the participants was Barry Beyerstein, a skeptical psychologist from Simon Fraser University. Other members of the panel included attorney Robert Kuhn, the program's host; anthropologist Marilyn Schlitz, who at the time was the research director of the Institute of Noetic Sciences; and psychologist Charles Tart, a well-known researcher of psi phenomena and a founder of transpersonal psychology. We were discussing the issue of replication of psi effects in the laboratory when the following exchange took place:

BARRY BEYERSTEIN: My trouble is that for the last twenty years I've been asking my psychology students to try replicating classic parapsychological experiments, without any positive results whatsoever. Since I have a random-number generator in my lab, other people from the community would come to ask my help in conducting ESP-type experiments. I've had psychics try to beat my random-number generator.

ROBERT KUHN: How have they done?

BARRY BEYERSTEIN: Zip. Nothing. I just can't get any replication in these things. . . .

ME: Are you claiming that you *never* get significant results?

BARRY BEYERSTEIN: I'm saying [I get] nothing more than chance would predict.

ME: OK, but you're getting a distribution of results, some of which are positive and some negative?

BARRY BEYERSTEIN: Individual trials and even individual persons may produce skewed results. If you run the random-number generator a hundred times, five of them, on average, will come out above chance. So the results match our statistical predictions for random behavior. . . . I like to take students who come to me because they want to prove me wrong. I give them the equipment, send them off, and say, "OK, if it's bad vibes from me, fine—I'll be gone." Some of these students have actually refused to give me their data, because they were so embarrassed when nothing nonrandom happened.

After the on-air portion of the program, I asked Beyerstein how he knew that his students' results were so poor given that they didn't share the data with him. I also asked if he had kept track of the twenty years' worth of failed experiments he claimed his students had conducted. He replied that he did not keep records of the experiments. So I pressed him to explain why he was so confident that the overall results were "zip," especially given what we have learned from meta-analysis—a popular method of analyzing the combined results of many similar experiments—where small but systematic effects in the same direction can compound into an extremely strong overall body of evidence. He had no response.

I could see from his reaction that it's uncomfortable to imagine that your deeply held beliefs might be wrong, especially when you're a professor who has professed those beliefs for years. But it doesn't take much effort or training to appreciate that there's a difference between belief in fairy tales and rigorously controlled scientific experiments.[110]

For example, Keith Stanovich's psychology textbook lists paranormal phenomena as "telepathy, clairvoyance, psychokinesis, precognition, reincarnation, biorhythms, astral projection, pyramid power, plant communication, and psychic surgery" (p. 186).[118] All these items are perfectly amenable to scientific inquiry, but so far only a few have been systematically investigated. Education may benefit by teaching students to avoid knee-jerk negative reactions to topics just because they seem peculiar and instead to evaluate what the evidence actually says. If there's no body of systematic scientific evidence to rely upon (e.g., for the viability of "pyramid power"), then we can't say much about that topic yet. But when there is evidence (as with several classes of psychic phenomena), then students should learn how to evaluate it.

Professors often give lip service to the importance of teaching critical thinking skills, but in practice most of that lip is arrogant and dismissive.

Another reason that the paranormal gets a bad rap is that professors are unaware of the evidence because their professors, and their professors before them, kept repeating that there wasn't anything worth paying attention to.[120] When something is repeated often enough, the lie takes on a life of its own. Political propagandists and advertising agencies have long capitalized on this fact.

Still another reason given by psychologists is that beliefs in phenomena "such as astrology and psychic powers share a common basis, namely a *violation of basic limiting principles of science*,"[121] or similarly, that such beliefs conflict with "current theories in physics."[122] What are these "basic limiting principles of science"? The phrase was introduced by philosopher C. D. Broad in a 1949 article.[123] He wrote:

> There are certain limiting principles which we unhesitatingly take for granted as the framework within which all our practical activities and our scientific theories are confined. Some of these seem to be self-evident. Others are so overwhelmingly supported by all the empirical facts which fall within the range of ordinary experience and the scientific elaborations of it (including under this heading orthodox psychology) that it hardly enters our heads to question them. Let us call these *Basic Limiting Principles*. Now psychical research is concerned with alleged events which seem *prima facie* to conflict with one or more of these principles.[123]

Broad then presents these principles in four general categories. The first is that it is impossible to have an effect before a cause. This rules out any form of retrocausation, including precognition. The second, that direct mind-matter interactions are impossible, except perhaps if the mind changes brain activity. This rules out any form of psychokinesis, including effects of prayer or other forms of mental healing from a distance. The third, that mental events depend completely on the brain, ruling out the possibility of out-of-body states or of survival of consciousness after bodily death. The fourth, that it is impossible to gain information about anything that occurs outside the body except through means conveyed by the ordinary senses. This rules out clairvoyance or remote viewing.

After reviewing the evidence for psychic abilities observed in laboratory studies, which Broad considered to be "facts which have been established to the satisfaction of everyone who is familiar with the evidence and is not the victim of invincible prejudice," he concluded:

> To sum up about the implications of the various kinds of paranormal cognition. It seems plain that they call for very radical changes in a number of our basic limiting principles.[123]

In other words, teachers who rely on Broad's limiting principles to discount the plausibility of psychic phenomena do not realize that the reason Broad stated those principles in the first place was to argue, based on the empirical evidence, that a major change in such "self-evident" principles was *required*. That was over a half century ago. The evidence is much stronger today.

The Wired Brain

A different approach to understanding why people believe in psychic phenomena, one that does not assume the presence of defective reasoning or some other lack of mental hygiene, is that the brain is simply wired to believe. Sharon Begley, a *Newsweek* science reporter, writes:

> That we are suckers for weird beliefs reflects the fact that the brain systems that allow and even encourage them "evolved

for other things," says James Griffith, a psychiatrist and neurologist at George Washington University. A bundle of neurons in the superior parietal lobe, a region toward the top and rear of the brain, for instance, distinguishes where your body ends and the material world begins. Without it, you couldn't navigate through a door frame.

But other areas of the brain, including the thinking regions in the frontal lobes, sometimes send "turn off!" signals to this structure, such as when we are falling asleep or when we feel physical communion with another person (that's a euphemism for sex). During intense prayer or meditation, brain-imaging studies show, the [superior parietal lobe] is also especially quiet. Unable to find the dividing line between self and world, the brain adapts by experiencing a sense of holism and connectedness. You feel a part of something larger than yourself.[124]

Notice that this explanation assumes, without question, that the sense of connection is a brain-generated hallucination. Begley didn't think it was worthwhile to ask whether these experiences *might* be real. As we shall see later, many experiments have investigated this question and they've found that some form of holistic connections are indeed quite real. You will not find this reported in *Newsweek*.

The Incredulous Brain

Let's examine this issue about "the believing brain" in more detail. A number of authors have expanded upon the idea that we believe in strange things because we are hardwired to do so, and that this brain-centric mechanism explains why so many people believe in psychic phenomena. Two books will serve for our discussion. One is by an academic psychologist, Richard Wiseman, and the other by a publisher of a skeptical magazine, Michael Shermer. Both are outspoken defenders of the skeptical faith.

Shermer's book *The Believing Brain* is subtitled *How We Construct Beliefs and Reinforce Them as Truths*, by which he means why *you* are silly enough to believe in ghosts, gods, the wrong flavor of politics, and outlandish conspiracy theories, but not him.[125] Wiseman's book *Paranormality* is subtitled *Why We See What Isn't There*, again meaning why *you* have delusional beliefs in ghosts, psychics, mind over matter, and precognition, but not him.[120]

Wiseman's thesis is that it is easy to be fooled into believing things that are not so, sometimes intentionally and sometimes inadvertently.[120] This is undoubtedly correct. We are all prone to remembering a few amazing coincidences in our lives and forgetting the much larger number of seemingly unrelated, mundane events. For example, one day while driving home from work I found myself thinking, out of the blue, about how much I liked spaghetti with marinara sauce. I knew we didn't have spaghetti at home, but that didn't stop my stomach from dreaming about spaghetti. When I arrived home, the first thing my wife said was that she bought me spaghetti with marinara sauce. I don't recall that she had ever done that before, and we hadn't communicated during the day at all. Coincidence?

Perhaps. We are poor estimators of the probability of events, and we are quick to jump at exciting paranormal reasons for strange bumps in the night when more boring explanations might suffice. In Wiseman's concluding chapter, he raised the question of why we evolved to "experience the impossible," by which he means anything that carries a whiff of the paranormal.

He concluded that it's based on the evolutionary pressure for us to be able to quickly identify patterns in randomness. If we didn't see the tiger hiding in the bush, we wouldn't be here today. And if we mistakenly saw a tiger when there wasn't one, we might be frightened for a second, but on the whole no harm would be done. This asymmetry leads us to see and believe in spooky things that aren't there. Of course, that very same superior pattern-recognition ability can also lead us to see and believe in things that actually *are* there, which Wiseman doesn't mention.

Shermer's book delves into more detail on Wiseman's question of "why we evolved this way." Shermer writes that he was once an unwavering Christian fundamentalist; now he's an equally unwavering atheist materialist. Among other things, this means he believes his mind is a brain-generated illusion, and that he and everyone else are ultimately mindless. I do not say this as a jab. It's simply the orthodox neuroscience worldview, in which all subjective experience is due solely to the firing of brain neurons.

Like Wiseman, Shermer posits that the brain is a "belief engine" that is hardwired to look for patterns. It assigns those patterns meaning, intention, and agency, and with a bit of reinforcement the patterns quickly harden into tenaciously held beliefs. The brain enjoys finding evidence that confirms its beliefs, which ultimately leads to a comfortably closed cycle in which what the brain believes determines what it is able to see, and that in turn reinforces what it believes. The smarter the brain, the more capable it is in rationalizing its beliefs, independent of whether those beliefs were obtained by what Shermer calls "nonsmart" reasons.

The credible portion of these books are the sections that discuss how we create and sustain strongly held beliefs. But things go terribly wrong when the authors then use these ideas to explain away paranormal beliefs. Both authors readily identify biases in others but fail to see them in themselves. This leads them to report information that supports their case and to ignore the rest. They also fail to address the "sunk cost bias," described by Upton Sinclair as, "It's difficult to get a man to understand something when his job depends on not understanding it."

Let's consider an example from Wiseman's book *Paranormality*. The book opens with an account of how he learned about "Jaytee," a dog who reportedly displayed a telepathic connection with his human companion, a woman named Pam Smart. Whenever Pam was returning home, her parents noticed that the dog went to a certain spot near the front window of the house and patiently waited for her. Otherwise the dog spent hardly any time at that location.

Wiseman described a series of experiments he conducted to see if Jaytee was genuinely telepathic, and he stated that he found no evidence for it. This story provided his book with an opening gambit to explain how easy it is for ordinary folks to fool themselves into thinking that something as obviously weird as dog telepathy was real. Readers who hadn't previously encountered this story would find it an amusing tale that soundly debunked the idea that some dogs knew when their human companions were returning home.

But for those who do know the full story, there's a conspicuous omission. In brief, British biologist Rupert Sheldrake first tested Smart's claim about Jaytee. Sheldrake eventually conducted some two hundred test sessions with the dog that demonstrated to very high levels of certainty that Jaytee did indeed anticipate Smart's return in ways that could not be explained through ordinary means.[126] By contrast, Wiseman conducted a mere four test sessions and yet he claimed that there was no evidence at all to support Jaytee's ability. Ignoring Sheldrake's much larger database was questionable, but even more troubling was the fact that Wiseman obtained exactly the same pattern of results as Sheldrake did, which he failed to mention.

In 2002, I asked Sheldrake if I could see the data from his and Wiseman's experiments, and he kindly supplied it.[127] I was able to confirm that the results were indeed strongly in favor of Sheldrake's conclusions, namely that Jaytee's behavior changed dramatically when Pam was returning home from many miles away, and when the signal to return was determined randomly and was unknown to anyone near Jaytee. Sheldrake's test designs had evolved to exclude all known loopholes, and the observed results remained the same. Nothing about this truly exceptional side of the story is mentioned in Wiseman's book.

There are other omissions, but the most outrageous is the fact that every single one of the targets of Wiseman's debunking—from psychics to mediums to precognition in dreams—has been thoroughly tested under controlled laboratory conditions. And unlike naive psychology professors who don't know any better because they're just repeating what they've been told, Wiseman obtained his doctorate under the auspices of the Koestler Unit of Parapsychology at the University of Edinburgh, one of the few places in the academic world where this sort of information is not ignored.

And indeed, in 2008 Wiseman confessed that in his opinion the accumulated scientific evidence for psychic phenomena was so persuasive that in an interview with the British newspaper the *Daily Mail* he provided an unexpected admission: "By the standards of any other area of science[,] remote viewing is proven. . . ."[128]

The import of this statement cannot be overstated.

A prominent skeptic of all things psychic, holder of Britain's only "Professorship for the Public Understanding of Psychology," a member of the Magic Circle (a London-based organization for stage magicians), and the self-described "most followed British psychologist on Twitter," Wiseman admitted that he believes psychic functioning has been scientifically proven. He later clarified that he meant to say not just remote viewing (i.e., clairvoyance) was proven, but that *all psi phenomena* "meet the usual standards for a normal claim," and are thus proven by scientific standards.

Despite this, Wiseman doesn't believe in psi.[129] Why not? Because like many skeptics he also believes that when it comes to assessment of unusual claims, higher standards of evidence are required. So for Wiseman psi would be proven if it were a normal claim, but for a supernormal claim it's just not good enough.

This may sound reasonable because surprising claims are always more difficult to believe than unsurprising claims. But it also masks a problem: The meaning of extraordinary is always in the eye of the beholder. For a Western-trained academic psychologist, the mere existence of, say, telepathy would be considered supernormal and thus wildly extraordinary. But for an experienced yogi, it's just a boringly normal minor siddhi. The skeptical psychologist, not having the benefit of thousands of hours of practice in yoga and meditation, requires repeatable, rigorously obtained experimental data showing odds against chance of a gazillion to one. The yogi merely requires his own experience.

And even in the face of substantial, repeatable evidence, skeptics persist in arguing that maybe those experiments are flawed in some unknown way. Maybe there's something fundamentally wrong with our methodologies. Maybe gremlins did it. Maybe . . . Beyond the endless series of maybes, why did Wiseman leave the revelation of "psi is proven" (if it were a normal phenomenon) out of his book? Perhaps Shermer's book *The Believing Brain* can help us to understand.

Unfortunately, Shermer makes things worse. While reading *The Believing Brain*, I kept stumbling over minor and major errors. As an example of a minor problem, Shermer implies that piercing one's arm with a ten-inch-long skewer, feeling no pain, and producing only a drop of blood is explainable only as a magician's trick (i.e., the needle only appears to pierce the arm). Perhaps he hadn't heard about Sufi rapid wound healing,[130] or of the anesthetizing effects of hypnosis, both of which dramatically demonstrate that people in the right state of mind, a religious ritual in the first case and a deep trance in the second, can indeed pierce their arm, tongue, cheek, or abdomen, with no pain and minimal or no blood loss, and then exhibit incredibly fast healing of the wounds. This may be surprising, but it is also an observable fact.

Major problems include Shermer's reaction to the renowned physicist Freeman Dyson, who to Shermer's distress endorsed the reality of psychic abilities in a book review published in the *New York Times*.[131] In an anti-Dyson screed published in *Scientific American*, Shermer asserted, "Either people can read each other's minds (or ESP cards), or they can't. Science has unequivocally demonstrated that they can't— Q.E.D." (p. 32).[132]

Really? As we'll see, scientific tests have actually demonstrated exactly the opposite conclusion. Even Wiseman agrees with that.

When a distinguished but elderly scientist states that something is possible, he is almost certainly right. When he states that something is impossible, he is very probably wrong.

—*Arthur C. Clarke's first law of prediction*

When a famous physicist endorses psychic ability in a prominent public forum, it upsets the scientific orthodoxy. A common reaction that is used when the offending believer is a respected but aging scientist is to question his or her mental faculties. It is acceptable to imagine that one can believe in ESP if one has dementia, but not if the mind is sound. So we should not be surprised to read John Horgan's words in a *Scientific American* blog:

> Much more damaging to Dyson's credibility, however, is his belief in extrasensory perception, sometimes called "psi." Dyson disclosed this belief in his essay "One in a Million" in the March 25, 2004, *New York Review of Books,* which discussed a book about ESP. His family, Dyson revealed, included two "fervent believers in paranormal phenomena," a grandmother who was a "notorious and successful faith healer" and a cousin who edited the *Journal of the Society for Psychical Research.*
>
> Dyson proposed that "paranormal phenomena are real but lie outside the limits of science." No one has produced empirical proof of psi, he conjectured, because it tends to occur under conditions of "strong emotion and stress," which are "inherently incompatible with controlled scientific procedures. . . ."[133]

Now we are faced with a double whammy. I have good reason to agree with Dyson's belief, but we come to that belief from entirely different directions. Dyson bases his belief on his family history, not on the scientific data. I have no familial reasons to believe in ESP, but I do find the scientific data to be persuasive.

However, because Dyson is not familiar with the empirical data, he is wrong in believing that conditions of strong emotion and stress are incompatible with controlled scientific procedures. Perhaps we can forgive him, being a physicist, for not realizing that the study of emotion, and effective means of producing it under controlled conditions, is very well developed within the disciplines of psychology and psychophysiology. Later I describe an experiment that intentionally modulated emotion to explore an unconscious form of precognition. That technique produces repeatable, surprisingly robust effects.

• • •

Returning to Shermer's errors, he asserts that when an experimenter and remote viewer are both blinded to the target, "psychic powers vanish." For over a century investigators studying psychic effects have developed protocols to explicitly avoid this obvious bias, as well as many more that are not so obvious. As we'll see, evidence for psychic abilities definitively does not vanish under these conditions.

Then he cites a study conducted by anthropologist Marilyn Schlitz, former president of the Institute of Noetic Sciences, who collaborated with Richard Wiseman on laboratory studies of the feeling-of-being-stared-at. Schlitz obtained significant results indicating that people could sense when they were being stared at, but Wiseman did not. Shermer interprets this as an "experimenter bias problem," apparently unaware that the two investigators were specifically studying the effect of the experimenter by working in the same lab at the same time, using the same procedures and equipment, the same participant population, and the same analyses. They still obtained different results.[134] Shermer continued:

> Scientists have now conclusively demonstrated what typically happens in research in which one subject tries to determine or anticipate the thoughts or actions of a second subject using paranormal means. . . . When the second subject is instructed to randomly perform some task . . . the sequence is not going to be random. Over time the second subject will develop a predictable pattern that the first subject will unconsciously learn.[125]

This might be true if experiments were conducted that way. But researchers are well aware that people do not act randomly, and as a result such experiments have not been conducted this way *for over a century.*

There is no need to belabor this exercise. I agree that beliefs distort what we can perceive, beliefs are inevitable, and science is the best method devised so far to slice through the distortions generated by our beliefs. But given these two authors' mistakes, we are obliged to reconsider the plight of the poor professional skeptics. They understand, intellectually at least, that beliefs bias perception. But they are incapable of transcending their own beliefs when confronted by discomforting data.

What happens when I turn the glare of this analysis onto my own position? The power of belief is such that I too am undoubtedly blind to some things that I prefer not to see. But there's a difference between where I stand and the hard-bitten skeptic. I claim that the cumulative experimental evidence is strong enough to make a case that genuine connections do exist between people, and between people and objects at a distance.

If my belief based on evidence is true, even to the slightest degree, then the skeptical house of cards falls apart. The skeptic's position, after all, is that absolutely *nothing* interesting is going on, despite admissions (in Wiseman's case) that the cumulative evidence actually is persuasive. Given this asymmetry, the professional skeptic must continue to deny or ignore all positive evidence because otherwise the "sunk cost" of an entire career is at stake. That's a heavy burden to bear when the evidence just keeps on getting stronger.

Personality

Belief is a powerful modulator of what we allow ourselves to see; that includes not just seeing the evidence for psi, but actual psi performance in experimental tasks. In 1946, psychologists Gertrude Schmeidler and Gardner Murphy tested whether people who believed in ESP would get different scores on simple symbol-guessing tests than those who did not believe. They found in each of six series of tests that those who believed scored higher than the others, with odds against chance of 33,000 to 1.[135] This "sheep-goat" effect, the sheep being the believers and the goats the disbelievers, has been repeated many times.

In 1993, psychologist Tony Lawrence, a graduate student at the University of Edinburgh at the time, conducted a meta-analysis of all sheep-goat forced-choice psi experiences conducted between 1943 and 1993. He found 73 publications reported by 37 different investigators, involving over 685,000 guesses produced by 4,500 participants. The overall results showed that believers performed better than disbelievers with odds against chance greater than a trillion to one.[136]

Belief is determined by personal experience, but it is also mediated by natural predilections. Some people are just naturally more open to contemplating new ideas or are more comfortable with intuitive rather than logical ways of thinking. Psychologists have found that this sort of person tends to believe in mysticism and in psychic experiences. Australian psychologist Michael Thalbourne proposed the word *transliminality* to describe the tendency in these people for their unconscious impressions to easily emerge into their consciousness.[137]

In the popular Myers-Briggs Type Inventory, or MBTI, personality test, there are four basic types of personality dimensions: Extrovert-Introvert, Sensing-Intuition, Thinking-Feeling, and Perceiving-Judging. The meaning of the fourth dimension is not immediately obvious; it refers to the need for order versus spontaneity. Thus "perceiving" refers to a person who is comfortable with spontaneity, while "judging" refers to a person with a preference for planning and order.

People with strong intuition-feeling characteristics, or "NF" types, are known to have mystical sentiments and are naturally drawn to mysticism, the occult, meditation, psi research, and esoteric practices. Their polar opposites, the sensing-thinking or "ST" types, have no interest in these matters.

In a study designed to assist people who were grieving over lost loved ones, hospice chaplain Dianne Arcangel measured each person's Myers-Briggs Type Inventory to see if there were personality differences in people reporting after-death contact experiences.[138] She found that a whopping 96 percent of the intuitive-feeling participants reported some form of after-death contacts, whereas 100 percent of the sensing-thinking participants types did not.

Not surprisingly, sensing-thinking people tend to be focused on the here and now, the materialistic, and rational, logical ideas. Sensing-thinking-*judging* (STJ) types are interested in management, leadership and authority in hierarchical organizations, and in the use of power to control rather than in creative or novel ideas. The extroverted STJ person is most prominent in Western culture. When the Myers-Briggs Type Inventory was given to thousands of people in large organizations, 60 percent of the top executive positions had STJ personalities, and the proportion of STJ types increased as their management level increased. Only about 1 percent of top executives had the opposite, intuitive-feeling-perceiving, or NFP, personalities.[139]

This means there is an automatic bias toward materialistic and pragmatic interests among those who control funding and power in large organizations, including federal science agencies, and a gaping deficit in those who are interested in the mystical and intuitive. And that's why it isn't surprising that psi research cannot be found within large corporate, government, or academic programs. At least, not publicly.

Transcending the Taboo

Many scientists are convinced that mechanistic materialism as a doctrine is all that will ever be needed to explain everything in the universe, including consciousness. But there are signs that this confidence is crumbling. As anthropologist Terrance Deacon has said, "Even as our scientific tools have given us mastery over so much of the physical world around and within us, they have at the same time alienated us from these same realms. It is time to find our way home."[140]

One way this restlessness can be seen is through a flurry of books evangelizing the new atheism, which is essentially a deification of materialism. In reaction, there is another rash of books exploring how science supports spirituality,[54] arguments suggesting the end of materialism,[141] how dogma constrains scientific advancements,[142] reformations of assumptions about the mind-matter relationship,[140] and challenges to neuroscience's assumptions about the brain-mind relationship.[143]

In one of these books, cell biologist Robert Lanza proposed a concept that he called biocentrism, which questions the traditional understanding of reality "creating" the observer. Instead,

> the animal observer creates reality and not the other way around. This is not some minor tweak in worldview. Our entire education system in all disciplines, the construction of our language, and our socially accepted "givens"—those starting points in conversations—revolve around a bottom-line mindset that assumes a separate universe "out there" into which we have each individually arrived on a very temporary basis.
>
> It is further assumed that we accurately perceive this external pre-existing reality and play little or no role in its appearance. . . . [But] absent the act of seeing, thinking, hearing—in short, awareness in its myriad aspects—what have we got? We can believe and aver that there's a universe out there even if all living creatures were nonexistent, but this idea is merely a thought and a thought requires a thinking organism.[144] (p. 157)

As openness to novel ideas about consciousness and reality continues to proliferate among scientists, a refreshing tolerance is also developing for a serious reconsideration of the supernormal. This would have pleased the yogis and sages, who recognized that someday science might have the capacity to advance our understanding of spirituality.

Yogananda wrote about witnessing the siddhis, but he also noted, "We must bear in mind that what was mystical a thousand years ago is no longer so, and what is mysterious now may become lawfully intelligible a hundred years hence. It is the Infinite, the Ocean of Power, that is at the back of all manifestations" (p. 322).[26] Likewise, Swami Rama wrote, "All the spiritual practices should be verified scientifically if science has the capacity to do so" (p. 3550).[145] And then, after describing the experience of witnessing a yogi turn his body into a hazy cloud and then back again into solid form, he added:

> I feel that the world should know that such sages exist, and the researchers should start researching such secret signs. Miracles like this show that a human being has such abilities. . . . I do not profess or claim that such siddhis are essential for self-enlightenment, but I want to say that human potentials are immense, and as the physical scientists are exploring the external world, the genuine yogis should not stop exploring the inner abilities and potentials.[145] (p. 3126)

The Dalai Lama agrees that the combination of modern and ancient methods for exploring reality are both necessary to form a better understanding, and not to throw spirituality away:

> Today, modern science, not through meditation, nor through logic, but through actual experiment, is discovering realities which sometimes go contrary to the scriptures. So in some cases modern science is even more powerful than ancient logic and meditation. But still, you see, I think even science has some limitations. Because there must be some other, more profound levels of reality which cannot be reached by ordinary perception or ordinary consciousness.[146] (p. 18)

Summary

Beliefs determine what we can see. People trained within the scientific and scholarly worldviews are taught that supernormal capacities are impossible, so mysticism and miracles are hardly ever taken seriously in academia, even among scholars in the history of religion. Such topics are fun to contemplate for entertainment purposes, or as a way to study primitive beliefs, but surely they're not *real*. As a result they're not included in the scientific story of reality that we've been taught in school, which is based on a few centuries of careful objective investigation.

What do worldviews that were developed over *thousands* of years of diligent subjective investigation tell us?

CHAPTER 6

Yoga Sutras

The quest to define the limits of the physically possible is, of course, a legitimate and indeed necessary scientific enterprise. But we have to take care that we really have surveyed all relevant possibilities. The history of science is littered with the wreckage of failed impossibility "proofs." [John] Bell has warned us that "what is usually demonstrated by impossibility proofs is a lack of imagination."

—*Yakir Aharonov*[147]

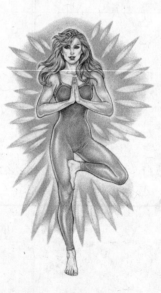

Yoga is not a religion in any traditional sense. It has no prescribed dogma, and it is practiced cheerfully by theists and atheists alike. In the West today, two components of traditional yoga have become part of popular culture: physical fitness through stretching and flexibility (in Sanskrit this is called *asana*), and mental fitness through the practice of meditation (*dhyana*). Those two aspects of yogic practice are what most Westerners know about yoga. But for thousands of years, the essential goal of yoga was to achieve states of insight that revealed the true nature of Reality, before personal biases and cultural expectations have a chance to distort our perceptions.

Yoga is often associated with Hinduism, but it predates Hinduism by centuries, possibly by millennia, and it is also closely associated with the histories of Jainism and Buddhism. While the origins of yoga remain shrouded in the oral histories of the ancient past, most scholars agree that it can be traced to between three thousand and five thousand years ago. Stone carvings depicting figures that appear to be in traditional yoga positions (like sitting in a lotus position) have been found in archaeological sites in the Indus Valley in India dating back to at least five thousand years.[148]

With prehistoric origins, it isn't possible in one chapter to thoroughly review yoga's many rich variations, techniques, and philosophies. I will present just enough of a sketch to provide a context for our focus on the siddhis.

In addition, yoga isn't the only practice with the lofty goal of enlightenment. Virtually all the various mystery schools and meditation systems are about exploring and transcending the boundary between the personal and the universal. A universal "Self" is personalized in religious traditions as God, Allah, Jehovah, Krishna, or by innumerable other names. But the Self can also be regarded as wholly *impersonal*. As Albert Einstein put it,

> The religious geniuses of all ages have been distinguished by
> this kind of religious feeling, which knows no dogma and no

God conceived in man's image; so that there can be no Church whose central teachings are based on it. Hence it is precisely among the heretics of every age that we find men who were filled with the highest kind of religious feeling and were in many cases regarded by their contemporaries as Atheists, sometimes also as saints.[81] (p. 21)

Regardless of how this higher sense of awareness is experienced, it has the power to transform the limited, localized, everyday sense of self into something remarkable. British psychologist David Fontana described the transformation as "an expansion which is not annihilation, not a loss of individuality, but a reality in which the distinction between individuality and unity, as between all opposites, not only disappears but is seen never truly to have existed" (p. 213).[149] That is, one awakens, as though everything experienced before then was in a dream.

Yoga Sutras

Before blogs and social networks, knowledge was preserved through oral traditions and practical presentations. And unlike revealed teachings, which rapidly become distorted or embellished as stories are told and retold, yoga was more like learning a practical trade instead of a set of philosophical doctrines. As such, the wisdom of countless generations of sages who developed yoga may be better preserved than other forms of historical lore.

What is now sometimes referred to as Classical yoga follows the principles outlined in a manuscript called the *Yoga Sutras*, written by the Indian sage Patanjali about two thousand years ago.[60] The Sanskrit word *sutra* is a cognate of *suture,* or thread. Patanjali's work is considered one of the first written documents to collect the threads of the oral history of yoga into a coherent tapestry. That the *Yoga Sutras* are still carefully studied and commented upon today is a testament to Patanjali's skill and to the wisdom of that oral tradition.[18]

The *Yoga Sutras* consist of four short books called *padas*, consisting of 196 aphorisms. Because the original is in Sanskrit, translation into English leaves plenty of room for interpretation. Dozens of books and hundreds of papers have been written with varying opinions on how to interpret the *Yoga Sutras*. In discussing what these books are about, I will for the most part avoid debates about which underlying philosophical system Patanjali may have had in mind when he wrote the *Sutras*, and I will also sidestep many of the other subtleties that have sustained the interests of Vedic philosophers and historians for centuries.

The four parts of the *Yoga Sutras* are (1) *Samadhi Pada*, a list of 51 aphorisms about the nature of meditative absorption; (2) *Sadhana Pada*, 55 aphorisms on the practice of yoga; (3) *Vibhuti Pada*, 56 aphorisms on the extraordinary abilities, the siddhis, that one encounters along the yogic path; and (4) *Kaivalya Pada*, 34 aphorisms about the goal of yoga—liberation. In a nutshell, the *Yoga Sutras* teach that to achieve enlightenment one must master two principal skills: The first is dispassion (in Sanskrit this is termed *vairagya*) and the second is absorption through a deep meditative state called *samadhi*.

Samadhi Pada

The very first sutra is the exemplar of pithiness: *Samadhi Pada* I.1: *Atha yoga-anushasanam*, which translates to "Now commences the exposition of Yoga." That's the ancient Sanskrit version of an entire introductory chapter. The one-sentence introduction may have meant that Patanjali knew exactly what he wanted to say, so he honed each sutra down to its bare essence (likely), or that the printing press wasn't invented yet and books had to be copied by hand, so the shorter the better (also likely).

In this first chapter, Patanjali describes the nature and purpose of *samadhi*, a state of deep meditative absorption. Being able to achieve and sustain samadhi at will is the key goal of traditional yoga practice, and the basic method for doing this is captured in the second sutra: *Yogas-citta-vritti-nirodha,* which may be translated as "Yoga is the restraint of mental distractions," or "Yoga is the restraint of the modifications of the mind-stuff."[17] When that state is fully achieved, it is accompanied by an experience of overwhelming bliss or ecstasy. As yoga scholar Georg Feuerstein put it:

> What all branches and schools of Yoga have in common [is] a state of being, or consciousness, that is truly extraordinary. One ancient Yoga authority captures this essential orientation in the following equation: "Yoga is ecstasy." In this context, the Sanskrit word for "ecstasy" is samadhi. The word samadhi . . . is composed of the prefixes *sam* (similar to the Latin syn) and *a,* followed by the verbal root *dha* ("to place, put") in its feminine form *dhi.* The literal meaning of the term is thus "placing, putting together." What is put together, or unified, is the conscious subject and its object or objects. Samadhi is both the technique of unifying consciousness and the resulting state of ecstatic union with the object of contemplation.[60] (p. 11)

The third sutra is *Tada drashthuh svarupe 'vasthanam,* or "Then the Seer appears," meaning that after the whirls and distractions of consciousness are successfully constrained and mental distractions settle down, then the transcendental Self appears.

That's all there is to it. Simple!

Alas, not so easy.

Despite breathless ads hawking amazing audio programs and electronic gadgets guaranteeing that you'll be meditating like a Buddhist monk in only thirty minutes, achieving this state is not so simple. Like all meditative states, samadhi has many layers of subtleties, each more refined than the last. In the Buddhist meditative tradition, for example, one can begin to develop the siddhis (known as *abbiññās* in Pali, the language of early Buddhism) only after mastering four levels of samadhi.[150]

Most people's minds are awash in a buzz of thoughts, worries, and desires. From that splintered mental state, which is reinforced by the necessities of daily life, samadhi sounds like a vacation to a Valium-scented fantasy island. Work, commuting, and chronic television violence are very effective at smothering the equanimity and silence necessary to develop and sustain samadhi. That's why when one seri-ously practices yoga at a traditional ashram (retreat center), there are no mundane distractions. No television, radio, iPod, cell phone, Inter-net, sugar, caffeine, spicy foods, clocks, and in some cases, no talking.

The ecstasy associated with the experience of samadhi might sound superficially similar to the momentary high achieved by smok-ing crack or shooting heroin. But while narcotics can blast the mind into a euphoric stupor, it doesn't take long before that route becomes horrifically grim, to say nothing of fleeting and a considerable drain on society. By contrast, the mind trained to sustain samadhi is focused, calm, and crystal clear, and the accompanying happiness doesn't fade or cost anything (other than maintaining a lifestyle that is probably much simpler than most Westerners are willing to adopt).

The modern sophisticate has been taught to associate claims about "bliss" and "ecstasy" as starry-eyed New Age pabulum, or as a sign of taking one too many psychedelic drugs. But this is indeed the serious aspiration of yoga practice. It may not be simple to achieve this goal today, but nor was it all that easy even when Patanjali wrote the *Yoga Sutras*. Still, the sages insist it is achievable, and both history and con-temporary examples confirm that it is possible. These people smile and laugh too much. They burst with radiant health and generosity. We are suspicious of them.

They've been transformed out of the ordinary, and it shows.[151] As William James wrote in *The Varieties of Religious Experience*:

The yogi, or disciple, who has by these means overcome the obscurations of his lower nature sufficiently, enters into the condition termed samadhi, and comes face to face with facts which no instinct or reason can ever know.[83] (p. 293)

In spite of being ineffable, a great deal has been written about this profound experience because of its remarkable nature. According to philosopher of mysticism Robert Forman:

> In these brief moments, one is aware of no particular content for awareness, yet still remains awake inside. Not thinking of anything, aware of no feelings or perceptions, consciousness is left, very simply, alone. And because one is aware of no objects, we might describe the "structure" of experience at those moments as consciousness having *no* relationship between itself and its objects: consciousness alone, no content. But the second structure is both more complex and more interesting. For this is the first *permanent* shift, the first stage of enlightenment. . . . Consciousness now perceives itself in itself, and as *distinct from* and *witness to* everything one sees and does.[152] (p. 70)

Sadhana Pada

The second book of the *Yoga Sutras* describes the practice of yoga. The goal of practice is to break out of the destructive habits that distract the mind and in turn create suffering. Patanjali describes a method known as *ashtanga*, or the eightfold path.

PATH 1 is *Yama*, restraining from harmful behavior, or cautions on what behavior to avoid. This includes violence, injury, telling falsehoods, stealing, lasciviousness, greed, and in general adopting ethical and virtuous behavior.

PATH 2 is *Niyama*, developing beneficial behavior, or guidelines on what behaviors to encourage. This includes cleanliness, austerity, cultivating an attitude of gratitude and contentment, and being engaged in a disciplined practice of focus, devotion, and self-study.

PATH 3 is *Asana*, development of physical postures. These are designed to assist the mind and body in relaxing, through development of strength, steadiness, and flexibility. The purpose of the asanas is to prepare the body to comfortably withstand the rigors of long-term meditation.

PATH 4 is *Pranayama*, conscious breathing techniques. These further the mind's ability to focus, and they energize the body.

PATH 5 is *Pratyhara*, withdrawing from ordinary sensory perceptions and limiting focus to a single object of attention. Restricting one's attention frees the attention to concentrate on internal objects of attention, fostering even more tranquility of mind.

PATH 6 is *Dharana*, developing a steady, sustained concentration. The root word *dhri* in *dharana* means "to hold"; one holds attention on a single object of thought. This type of concentration is similar to that experienced during highly focused intellectual work.

PATH 7 is *Dhyana*, developing prolonged levels of concentration on an object, with deeper absorption and greater sustained alertness. This is sometimes referred to as meditation.

PATH 8 is *Samadhi*, unity or mystical absorption with an object of attention. In this state, distinctions between subject and object dissolve and one "becomes" the object of meditation. This awareness is frequently described as ecstatic. That is, it is a superaware state accompanied by intense, nonsensual pleasure.

Vibhuti Pada

The third book describes the siddhis, the supernormal powers achieved as a result of dedicated yoga practice. In fifty-six concise sutras, the siddhis are expressed as a natural side effect of gaining proficiency in sustaining a refined meditative state known as *samyama*. Samyama involves combining expertise in the last three steps of the eightfold path, *dharana* (concentration), *dhyana* (meditation), and *samadhi*, along with an object of attention.

The siddhis are presented with no fanfare and in a matter-of-fact way, simply as signposts that one should expect to encounter while on the yoga path. Until the recent rise of scientific authority, the siddhis were not even considered controversial. They were accepted as fact, along with many other types of miracles that are accepted on faith within most religions today. But because scientific theories have superseded religious doctrine as the arbiter of truth in the modern educated world, and because science has yet to develop adequate theoretical explanations for such phenomena, this creates a conflict, as Georg Feuerstein noted:

> Modern students are apt to dismiss the magical dimension of Yoga, but it is an integral aspect of yogic experience. Why else did Patanjali devote an entire chapter to paranormal powers (siddhi) in his Yoga-Sutra? . . . These powers are a natural by-product of the yogin's meditation practice. Yet, as Patanjali observes in his Yoga-Sutra (III.37), they are *accomplishments* only from the point of view of egoic consciousness.[60] (p. 40)

While the development of siddhis as a result of practicing samyama is an important part of yoga development, it is not a trivial affair, even for advanced yogis. As Swami Rama said,

> The science of raja yoga teaches *samyama*—inner transformation through *concentration, meditation, and samadhi*. During

this training I discovered that without living in silence for a considerable time, maintaining a deeper state of meditation is not possible.[145] (p. 3518)

In today's world, few of us have the passion or the resources to live in complete silence for extended periods, nor do most people have the natural talent to be able to sustain samyama at will even if they were lucky enough to live without any other responsibilities. The stereotyped image of a saddhu (holy man) wearing a loincloth in the austerity of a Himalayan cave is not that far from the kind of context that may be necessary to achieve expertise in the siddhis. And even if one did have the time, resources, and talent, Patanjali adds a warning. Swami Rama explains:

The third chapter of the *Yoga Sutras* explains many methods of attaining *siddhis* [powers], but these siddhis create stumbling blocks in the path of enlightenment. One person in millions does indeed have siddhis, but I have found that such people are often greedy, egotistical, and ignorant. . . . The miracles performed by Buddha, Christ, and other great sages were spontaneous and for a purpose. They were not performed with selfish motives or to create a sensation.[145] (p. 854)

In the next chapter we will explore the descriptions of the siddhis in more detail. For now, it is worth keeping in mind that among advanced yogis who knew from firsthand experience that the siddhis existed, they also understood that they were rare, they were seductive, and they could be, and often were, faked. This means that the concerns of conjurers and skeptics about the problems of fraudulent psychics and faked "powers" are nothing new. Nor is it new that some will take advantage of minor psychic talents to convince others that they have greater spiritual attainments or enlightenment than the average person. This is how cults are born.

Because the siddhis are so seductive, sages have repeatedly

reminded us to calm down and not dwell on them, because ultimately these abilities are only a reflection of the holistic nature of the universe. In particular, they say nothing about one's spiritual attainments. Swami Rama explains:

> These powers have nothing to do with spirituality. . . . Sometimes psychic powers develop; you start telling the fortunes of others, you start knowing things. These are all distractions. Do not allow them to obstruct your path. Too many people, including swamis, have wasted time and energy on such distractions. Anyone who wants to develop siddhis can do so and can demonstrate certain supernatural feats; but enlightenment is an entirely different matter.[145] (p. 873)

Kaivalya Pada

The last book of the *Yoga Sutras* is entitled *Kaivalya Pada*, or the book about liberation. In thirty-four sutras Patanjali describes *moksha*, the essential state of freedom that is the ultimate goal of yoga. This type of freedom refers to what happens when the mind loosens its grip on the world of appearances and experiences the world as it is, without the illusion of separation, without artificial hierarchies, and without dualistic concepts.

Many have waxed poetic about this state of spacious awareness, but ultimately verbal descriptions are inadequate, so any attempt to describe it is going to be unavoidably shallow and subject to cultural interpretation. Words reinforce the idea of separate concepts and temporal sequences, and yet the world as it is, as described by mystics throughout history, doesn't appear to be like that at all. On the other hand, words *are* powerful pointers to ideas (hence this book), so sometimes the right words in the right context may open doorways to mystical insights.

Summary

Patanjali's *Yoga Sutras* captures the core of the yogic tradition as it was practiced over countless preliterate millennia. Half of that book is devoted to discussions that challenge our very understanding of reality. Our language today is so dominated by sensory aspects of the objective world that when we are presented with deep subjective concepts touching upon the supernormal, or with subtleties associated with liberation of the mind, we are either stunned into silence or we reject that information as mere fantasy.

So enough said about the ineffable. Now let's look in more detail at the siddhis.

CHAPTER 7

The Siddhis

The whole history of science shows us that whenever the educated and scientific men of any age have denied the facts of other investigators on a priori grounds of absurdity or impossibility, the deniers have always been wrong.

—*Alfred Russell Wallace*

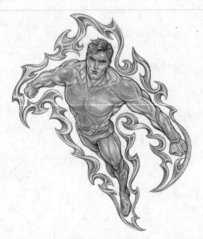

The *Yoga Sutras* provide a taxonomy of supernormal mental powers and a means of obtaining them. Today we would classify most of the siddhis as various forms of psychic, or psi, phenomena. Others might be called exceptionally precise means of controlling the mind-body relationship.

Samyama

Patanjali writes that the siddhis are attained after mastery of the last three steps of the eightfold path: the ability to simultaneously sustain concentration, meditation, and samadhi at will. "Sustained" in this context means holding a highly focused, unwavering, deeply absorbed meditative state—as opposed to obsessive mental chattering—*indefinitely*, if one so wishes.

Considering that beginning meditators may be satisfied to hold an unwavering focus for ten seconds, being able to do this for fifteen minutes at a time may seem incredible; for hours without end is practically incomprehensible. But that's the level of mental control said to be required to exercise the siddhis on demand.

And that's just the beginning. In the *Vibhuti Pada*, Book III of the *Yoga Sutras*, Patanjali writes that samyama might seem special to the uninitiated, but it is rather crude compared to where you really want to go. A translation of Sutra III.8 is: "In comparison to the seedless and unbound goal of enlightenment, samyama is to be viewed as a coarse and external component."[18] In other words, walking on water is trivial compared to what you really want to achieve, a state called *nirbija samadhi*, or samadhi without attenuation.

At this point, to prevent our heads from exploding after trying to imagine the intense practice and skill required to reach these states, let's return to the comparatively simple practice of samyama. As we do so, we will simply assume that after thousands of years of exploration, refinement, and discussion about these techniques, advanced yoga practitioners may have advanced far beyond what science is currently capable of confirming, and we'll leave it at that.

Depending on the nature of the object one is absorbed into during samyama, different siddhis are said to arise. This is not due to magical incantations, but a natural consequence of merging with the object of focus. For example, if one focuses on another person, in samyama one *becomes* the other person. The siddhi that arises is what we would call telepathy.

In the science fiction television series *Star Trek*, this practice was depicted as the Vulcan mind meld. Telepathy occurs in the mind meld (and in the siddhis) not because thoughts are transmitted from another person's mind to yours, but because while in samyama your mind breaks through the illusion of separation that tricks you into believing that you and the other person are different. In deep states of the absorptive mind meld, whether yogic or Vulcan, holistic reality reigns. You are no longer two people, but one and the same. The genius of *Star Trek* is that it is the dispassionate, hyperrational, deeply focused Vulcans who can achieve this state, and not the attention-deficit, emotionally uncontrolled humans.

As another example, in samyama one may focus on the processes of time, change, and transformation. The siddhi that arises is the simultaneous perception of the past, present, and the future. The idea that the present contains the past is common knowledge; we call this memory. The idea that the present is also influenced by the *future* may seem odd, but this quasi-teleological concept is accommodated within today's physics.[153] For example, in quantum theory the idea that the present is constrained by both the past *and* the future is respectable, but of greater importance, there is now experimental evidence supporting it, published in 2012 in the journal *Nature Physics*.[154] The originators of this concept are not mystics. They include physicist Yakir Aharonov, who was awarded the US National Medal of Science in 2010 and is regarded as one of the world's leading quantum theorists.[155, 156]

The future influencing the present might sound strange, but practically everything seems strange the moment we step outside of the everyday world and probe either the inner depths or the outer limits of reality. Likewise, the siddhis seem contrary to common sense only because they arise from depths of awareness that lie far beyond the common senses.

Taxonomy

Past, Present, and Future walk into a bar at the same time. It was tense.

Approximately twenty-five siddhis are listed in the third book of the *Yoga Sutras*. An exact number is difficult to pin down because the abilities may be interpreted in different ways, and there is some overlap. But it is possible to view all the siddhis as variations on three basic classes:

(1) EXCEPTIONAL mind-body control

(2) CLAIRVOYANCE, the ability to gain knowledge unbound by the ordinary constraints of space or time and without the use of the ordinary senses; includes precognition and telepathy

(3) PSYCHOKINESIS or mind-matter interaction, the ability of the mind to directly influence matter

Fifteen of the siddhis fall into the category of clairvoyance, four fit into the category of psychokinesis, and six in mind-body control. The siddhis listed here are in the order in which they appear in the *Yoga Sutras*:

PADA III. Sutra 16. (This will be abbreviated as III.16 in succeeding sutras.) *Knowledge of the past, present, and the future,* resulting from samyana on the nature of change. This is *clairvoyance* through time, commonly called *precognition* when the information obtained is from the future, or *retrocognition* if it is from the past (and is not simply memory).

III.17. Knowledge of the meaning of sounds produced by all beings, resulting from samyana on the "third ear," or the concept of sound, words, or hearing. This may be interpreted as a form of clairvoyance, or telepathy that extends beyond human minds and includes animals, insects, and other species. More generally it is known as clairaudience.

III.18. Knowledge of previous births and arising of future births, resulting from samyana on one's latent or inherited tendencies. This is clairvoyance on an aspect of consciousness that does not arise from the body and is sustained after bodily death. A similar siddhi is described in *Sadhana Pada* II.39, translated as "When non-greed is confirmed, a thorough illumination of the how and why of one's birth comes."[17]

III.19–20. Knowledge of minds, resulting from samyama on one's own mind or another's mind, both of which from a holistic perspective are part of the universal mind. We now call this telepathy.

III.21. Disappearance of the body from view, as a result of looking at the body with the inner eye. This is sometimes translated as the power of invisibility, because the Sanskrit aphorism contains words suggesting a "suspension of the coarse or limited projection of the body." But it may also be interpreted as the ability to perceive aspects of the body that are beyond the limited scope of the ordinary senses. In other words, we could interpret this as clairvoyance, or perhaps as psychokinesis.

III.22. Foreknowledge of birth, harm, or death, resulting from samyama on sequences of events in one's past and present. This again is a form of clairvoyance.

III.23. Loving-kindness in all, resulting from samyama on friendliness, compassion, or sympathetic joy. This can be interpreted to mean that when one is imbued with joy, that state may induce similar feelings in others. This may be interpreted as an unintentional or fieldlike form of psychokinesis.

III.24. Extraordinary strength, resulting from samyama on the concept of physical strength (the aphorism specifically mentions the strength of an elephant, which was undoubtedly the strongest creature in Patanjali's world), but it might also include mental, moral, or spiritual strength. This could be interpreted as an exceptional form of mind-body control or as a mind-matter interaction effect. Swami Satchidan-anda sums up this siddhi with the comment, "You can lighten yourself; you can make yourself heavy. It's all achieved by samyama. Do it; try it. Nice things will happen" (p. 188).[17]

III.25. Knowledge at a distance, resulting from samyama on the "inner light," which in Western esoteric terms is known as the "subtle body" or the "light body." This siddhi includes knowledge of hidden objects, or clairvoyance.

III.26. Knowledge of the outer universe, resulting from samyama on the solar principle, which could include the sun as a planetary body, or the concept of the solar plexus, one of the principal "subtle energy" centers or chakras in the human body. A more detailed translation of this sid-dhi would require a major diversion into esoteric yogic concepts where aspects of the human body, some physical and others more subtle, are mapped onto aspects of the cosmos. This arcane symbolism is outside the scope of the present book, so we may simply interpret this siddhi as clairvoyance of macroscopic objects and systems.

III.27–28. Knowledge of the inner universe, resulting from samyama on the lunar or *chandra* principle, or the "pole star." As with the previous sid-dhi, to avoid diverting our attention to esoteric lore that is not within the capacity of science to evaluate, we will interpret this as clairvoy-ance of microscopic objects and systems.

III.29. Knowledge of the composition and coordination of bodily energies, through samyama on the navel chakra or *manipura* chakra. This sid-dhi may be interpreted as an exceptional mind-body connection, or as a self-healing ability.

III.30. Liberation from hunger and thirst, through samyama on the throat. This siddhi is known as inedia within the Catholic tradition, or more popularly as breatharianism (living on breath alone, without food, and in extreme cases, without water).

III.31. Exceptional stability, balance, or health, through samyama on the *kurma nadi*, the root of the tongue. This siddhi refers to mind-body knowledge leading to exceptional health or self-healing.

III.32–36. Vision of higher beings, knowledge of everything that is knowable, knowing of the origins of all things, knowledge of the true self, through samyama on the crown of the head, intuition, the spiritual heart, the self, or the nature of existence. These siddhis are forms of refined clairvoyance.

III.37. Siddhis may appear to be supernormal, but they are normal. This is not a description of a siddhi, but rather a caution to avoid regarding the siddhis as unnatural or supernormal, as that could become a distraction to sustaining and deepening samadhi.

III.38. Influencing others. This siddhi suggests that a highly realized yogi who is adept with the previously described siddhis can not only know about others, but also influence them. This is related to the concept of *shaktipat*, the ability to transmit spiritual energy to others through one's gaze or presence. In laboratory jargon, this phenomenon is known as "distant mental interactions with living systems." It may be interpreted as a sort of field effect due to the rarified mental state that the yogi embodies, which acts like a radiating beacon that influences everyone in the vicinity. This siddhi is also related to a sutra described in the second book of the *Yoga Sutras, Sadhana Pada*. The translation of Sutra II.35 reads: "In the presence of one firmly established in nonviolence, all hostilities cease."[17]

III.39 and 42. Levitation, through samyama on the feeling of lightness. This siddhi is said to allow the yogi to float, hover, fly, or walk on water. It could be interpreted as a highly advanced form of psychokinesis.

III.40. Blazing radiance, through samyama on "inner fire," or inner energy. This has been interpreted in several ways, as possession of exceptional charisma, as an exceptional digestive ability that would allow one to eat huge amounts of food or withstand toxic substances without harm, or as exceptional control of bodily energies. We will interpret it as an exceptional form of mind-body control.

III.41. Clairaudience, through samyama on the area behind the ear. This siddhi allows one to hear the "conversations of the enlightened ones, the subtle mental conversations of others, the celestial music, and receive messages through the ether both awake or while asleep, as if they were spoken or whispered whether or not they exist through the medium of sound waves as such."[18] In other words, this is a refined form of clairvoyance or clairaudience.

III.43. Freedom from bodily awareness and temporal attachments. This could be interpreted as a state of perception from out-of-the-body, or as a form of clairvoyance.

III.44–45. Mastery over the elements, through samyama on the elements, enabling manipulation of matter, including the size, appearance, and condition of the body. Variations of these abilities include the fulfillment of any desire, or to create or destroy material manifestations; a highly refined version of psychokinesis.

III.46. Perfection of the body. This could be interpreted as a melding of exceptional mind-body control combined with psychokinesis. It would manifest in extreme cases as indefinite life extension, as incorruption of the body after physical death, perhaps as the "rainbow body" in Tibetan tradition, in which the corpse does not decay but rather slowly fades away and turns into colored lights.

This list covers Patanjali's classic siddhis; many other variations of these superpowers can be found in mystical texts from other traditions. They include bilocation (the ability to simultaneously appear in more than one location); the ability to move very fast or cover great distances in a short time; the ability to stay comfortably warm in extremely cold temperatures; the ability to suspend breathing or to hibernate indefinitely; the ability to bestow siddhis to others; the ability not to be harmed by fire; and the ability to change the weather.

Danger, Danger

Before we begin our scientific examination of the siddhis, it is noteworthy that Patanjali and others specifically highlighted the dangers of dwelling on the siddhis. Patanjali states in Sutra III.51 a warning that may be translated as:

Avoid invitations to display or identify with any accomplishments in yoga, including the siddhis, even if invited by a respected person, because this can reinforce one's sense of separate self, leading to ego, pride, and arrogance, and this becomes an impediment toward further spiritual unfoldment.[18]

There are many ways that this trap can manifest. If personal pride or greed causes one to be seduced by the ever-present challenge of proving one's abilities to skeptics, such as using psychic abilities to win a prize, then the power gained by that seduction is likely to corrupt the ethical restraints that are the very first lesson to learn on the eightfold path. That "power corrupts" is an unavoidable truth in human affairs, and the consequences of the fall in this case are profound because the goal of achieving enlightenment, which requires far more discipline than simply developing clairvoyance, is lost. Even if one does not personally identify with a siddhi, and instead attributes it to one's teacher or a particular lineage, the damage is done.

This means that from a scientific perspective it may be exceptionally difficult to find people who have achieved these rarified states *and* are willing to demonstrate them, because paradoxically they have reached those states precisely because they have *not* demonstrated them in public. When I have asked yogis who appear to have reached some level of mastery to participate in laboratory tests, only on very rare occasions have they agreed to do so. They usually performed remarkably well, but when I ask *how* they did it, or to do it again, they just smiled.

Fortunately, siddhis are not an all-or-nothing affair. They are not instant phase shifts that appear out of thin air, but rather they're stable versions of weaker effects that some people can demonstrate some of the time. If this were not so, then science would never have learned anything about the siddhis.

Proof?

A common complaint about the siddhis goes like this: If science has been studying these phenomena in a systematic way for over a century, then surely we should have settled the issue one way or the other by now. So the fact that the mere existence of these superpowers is still mired in controversy tells us that the siddhis don't exist.

This logic seems reasonable until one pays closer attention to the history of science. From the historical perspective this type of critique is simply a matter of impatience. For example, consider the case of magnetism.[157] One of the first recorded attempts to study magnetism in scientific terms was in 1269. Until then, everyone considered magnetism to be a magical phenomenon. But Peter Peregrinus, who was serving in the army of the king of Sicily, took a different tack. He decided to write down everything that was known at the time about lodestone (a natural magnetic ore) and how to make instruments using it.

Three hundred years later British scientist William Gilbert would again take up the challenge to explain magnetism in rational terms.

But another whole century would pass before scientists began to think of new ways to understand magnetism. Even then, it took the invention of highly abstract mathematical concepts before invisible forces like magnetism could even begin to be understood, and the truth is that even today we still don't understand *fundamentally* what magnetism actually *is*. We've learned a few tricks that describe how it behaves under certain circumstances, and we can make machines that take advantage of that knowledge. But that's all.

In any case, it took half a millennium for science to learn enough about magnetism to make it practically useful, and unlike psi, magnetism is easy to demonstrate. Similarly, physicists have developed models for how they think gravity works, but we still don't understand exactly what it *is*. Nor after many decades of intensive work by tens of thousands of scientists, funded to the tune of a trillion or more dollars, do we understand how to cure cancer. And no one has the slightest idea what consciousness is, despite it being the one and only thing any of us will ever personally know firsthand.

In sum, given that the number of mysteries in the universe that remain to be deciphered is practically infinite compared to the few trinkets of knowledge that we've discovered, it's astonishing that anyone could possibly argue that after a century of fits and starts we should already have a complete understanding of psi and the siddhis. Some progress has been made, but we've just begun.

Summary

The third book of the *Yoga Sutras* describes supernormal abilities in matter-of-fact terms. The siddhis are presented not as magical or divine gifts available to the lucky few but as natural consequences of intense meditation practice. Most of these abilities today would be regarded as variations of psychic phenomena, mainly variations of clairvoyance. But some of the siddhis stretch our sense of the possible beyond the breaking point. How should we regard such tales?

PART II

. . . To Modern Science

There is no source of deception in the investigation of nature which can compare with a fixed belief that certain kinds of phenomena are impossible.

—*William James*

Legends of supernormal powers are mind-boggling, complex, and confusing. Some of the claimed siddhis sound like pure fantasy; others seem more plausible. Must we take these legends on faith alone? Can they be measured and tested?

CHAPTER 8

Science and the Siddhis

If you take the word "normal" as characteristic of the norm or majority, then it is the superstitious and those who believe in ESP, ghosts and psychic phenomena who are normal. Most scientists and skeptics roll their eyes at such sleight of word, asserting that belief in anything for which there is no empirical evidence is a sign of mental pathology and not normalcy.

—*Sharon Begley,* Newsweek[124]

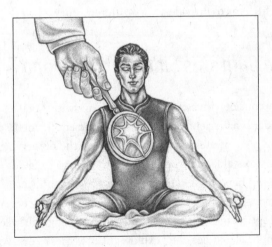

Is it pathological to believe in something with no empirical evidence? If so, then according to Sharon Begley, anyone who professes strong religious faith is mentally ill. With that gauntlet thrown down, no wonder theists and atheists are always at each other's throats. They both think their opponents are nuts.

But what about empirical proof of a mother's love for her child? We know something about the biochemical correlates of love, such as the presence of the "love hormone," oxytocin. We can also infer the presence of love by observing behavior. But when it comes down to proof of *felt* love, science is mum about mom. Science does not have ways of strictly objectifying first-person subjective experience. Only the "I" in you can do that.

In this chapter's opening quote, Sharon Begley was writing about a different kind of subjective experience—extrasensory perception, ESP. As she says, for some scientists merely mentioning this topic evokes uncontrollable spasms of eye rolling and deep sighing. But the phrase "no empirical evidence" is really just an excuse for dismissing the extraordinary. For those who don't feel threatened by novel ideas, there is plenty of evidence to be found, as we shall see. The question is how shall we reconcile the story of reality that science tells us with yogic lore, which seems to provide a very different story.

We Built This Siddhi on Rock and Roll

When we consider investigating the siddhis with science, we must first consider what science is *able* to study. Scientific methods are exceptionally good at measuring and modeling the observable world—from atoms to stars, and from bacteria to human behavior. If we are interested in phenomena where we want high confidence that what we're studying is *real*, rather than a mistake, a coincidence, or one or more perceptual biases, then we must turn to controlled laboratory experiments. Lab studies don't explore the raw, messy, everyday world at large. They investigate, usually with tight controls, artificially constrained versions of the real world.

In the lab, living cells are examined in petri dishes. Electrical activity in a person's brain is measured as he or she views various images. We may look for statistical shifts in the probability distributions of random events.

The price for gaining high confidence in these observations is that we have to narrow our focus and define the boundaries of what we're examining. In so doing, the effects that we end up seeing in the lab tend to be tiny as compared to what happens outside the lab. This is especially true when we're studying spontaneous human behavior.

In addition, scientific methods are not very effective in measuring purely *subjective* states. Psychological and physiological measurements allow us to infer what's happening in someone's conscious mind, and to a limited extent in their unconscious, but we cannot know it directly. Watching a yogi meditating, even with fancy brain-scanning machines, is not going to tell us much about what it's like to experience samadhi.

Fortunately, some siddhis are amenable to being studied under rigorously controlled laboratory conditions because they involve effects that *can* be objectively assessed. For example, we can examine whether siddhis involving clairvoyance or precognition provide genuine versus illusory information, we can test whether some extraordinary mind-body effects are verifiably real, and we can investigate whether mind-matter interactions exist.

We still face some important limitations—it isn't easy to find people with Buddha-level skills who are willing to come to the laboratory and display their gifts. As already mentioned, most esoteric practices explicitly warn against demonstrating these skills in public. So we are limited to investigating three classes of people: those who appear to be talented based on their prior performance in the lab, those who have some meditation and yoga practice, or—and this is how it ends up most of the time—volunteers who are unselected, untrained, and unskilled, but who are willing and able to participate in experiments.

Not being able to study the cream of the crop means the effects we see will probably be weak and sporadic. That means having to collect an enormous amount of data to gain confidence in the results. Fortunately there is also an advantage to studying ordinary people. If Joe Sixpack, our randomly picked "man off the street," can show weak but positive results in the lab, then it indicates that the siddhis are part of a spectrum of abilities that are broadly distributed across the population. It is much easier to accept the reality of a claimed skill if it turns out to be a basic human potential rather than an extreme idiosyncrasy that only a handful of people in the world possess.

I suspect that there are those among us who have high-functioning siddhis gained not through extensive meditation practice but through raw talent. Like Olympic athletes or Carnegie Hall musicians, these people are rare. Based on my experience in testing a wide range of participants in laboratory psi tests, I'd estimate that perhaps one in ten or a hundred thousand have exceptional skills comparable to the traditional siddhis.

The Really Big Siddhis

We must also consider whether to take the descriptions of the siddhis literally or as metaphors. Are siddhis about levitation or a complete mastery of mind over matter really true? Can diamonds literally appear from nowhere on mental command? Although there are historical accounts of these claims, and some contemporary gurus and psychics continue to make such claims, there are also plenty of people who are adept at faking them.

I've tested a few people who've made claims about exceptionally strong psychic effects and who swear that they are telling the truth. Not one of them was able to systematically demonstrate their claims under conditions that persuaded me that the effects were genuine. This doesn't necessarily mean that those claimants were telling bald-faced lies, or that they were delusional. To be charitable, some of the difficulty may be due to the tenuous nature of the phenomena. But Patanjali does not describe the siddhis as being feeble or unreliable. He writes that when samadhi is controlled, and samyama is achieved, these things happen. Period. They don't *sort of* happen depending on who's watching.

Two of the intermediate big siddhis, both involving supernormal control of the mind-body connection, do have some evidence: the ability to raise the body's core temperature to allow one to comfortably remain in snow and ice without clothing, and to no longer eat food.

The Ice Man

An amusing tradition in colder climes is the "Polar Bear" plunge, in which on New Year's Day tens of thousands of people dive into the icy ocean. This can be done safely for a few minutes provided that the body stays in motion and the person gets out of the water quickly. Under normal conditions, it is lethal to be exposed to icy water and freezing temperatures for more than a few minutes.

However, the Tibetan practice of *tummo* meditation, where *tummo* roughly means "inner fire," cultivates a mind-body connection in which extreme cold that would quickly kill an untrained person can be comfortably tolerated for minutes to hours. Tummo meditation may be related to the yogic concept of *kundalini* energy, a life-force energy said to circulate within the body. When properly focused, yogic lore says that it's possible to generate enough heat to sit still in freezing cold without harm. This claim was tested in Tibetan monks and confirmed by Harvard University's Herbert Benson and his colleagues.[158] While this ability is now known to be possible, the underlying mechanism remains a mystery.

The mystery deepened in recent years when Dutch athlete Wim Hof began to demonstrate truly extreme versions of bodily control through his practice of tummo.[100] In his book, *Becoming the Iceman*, Hof describes a series of increasingly remarkable feats, including running a full marathon at −4°F above the polar circle, on the snow, barefoot, and wearing just running shorts. He also holds the world's record for sitting still while submerged in ice water (for an hour and forty-four minutes), he climbed to the top of Mount Kilimanjaro wearing just his shorts, and if it were not for a foot injury he would have scaled Mount

Everest as well without oxygen tanks. Any of these feats would kill an average person.

Hof claims that everyone has the capacity to learn how to accomplish these feats (but perhaps not the will). This form of mental control of the body fits within the traditional description of the siddhis, for example in the *Yoga Sutras Pada* III.40: "blazing radiance." Research on Hof is beginning to confirm that these extreme forms of mind-body control are even more remarkable than just regulating body heat.

For example, as reported on the US National Institutes of Health website, Clinicaltrials.gov,[159] at Radboud University Nijmegen Medical Centre in the Netherlands, Hof was submerged in ice water for eighty minutes to study his body's response to the damage caused by the extreme cold. In another test he was injected with an endotoxin that creates an inflammatory response with fever, chills, and headache. The inflammation in Hof's body was measured through stress hormones in his blood. One of the study's authors, Peter Pickkers, said in an interview with the website ScienceDaily,

> After endotoxin administration, the increase of the stress hormone cortisol in Hof was much more pronounced compared to other healthy volunteers. We know that this hormone is released in response to increased autonomic nervous system activity and that it suppresses the immune response. In accordance, the levels of inflammatory mediators in Hof's blood were much lower. On average, Hof's immune response was decreased by 50 percent compared to other healthy volunteers. In addition, hardly any flu-like symptoms were observed. These results are definitely remarkable.[160]

Breatharianism

Breatharianism, the Qigong practice of *Bigu*, and the Catholic charism of inedia all involve the claim of living well without eating food. More extreme claims involve not drinking any liquid, either. The implication is that the human body can transmute ambient energy into nutrients, and through the practice of cultivating this ability one can live comfortably for as long as one wishes without food, and possibly without drinking water. This is described as a siddhi in the *Yoga Sutras* as *Pada* III.30: liberation from hunger and thirst.

This flies in the face of a substantial body of medical knowledge, which has established that the human body can last about five days without water, and a few weeks at most without food. Beyond that, you're dead. As a result, despite a host of historical examples of people lasting for years without eating, and sometimes without drinking, most nutritionists and biochemists regard such claims to be ridiculously impossible, and the people who make the claims—currently dozens to hundreds worldwide—to be seriously delusional. Some of those claimants may well be delusional. But all of them?

From my reading of this literature, there appear to be at least two contemporary cases that may cause us to pause and reconsider. The first is the case of the Indian sadhu Prahlad Jani. He describes a religious experience at age eleven when the Hindu goddess Amba appeared to him and told him that he would no longer have to eat food. He is said to have lived in a cave since the 1970s, and to have not eaten anything for most of his eighty-one years (as of 2012).

Jani was tested in 2003 and again in 2010 at Sterling Hospital in the western Indian city of Ahmedabad, by Dr. Sudhir Shah and his team. In the 2003 test, Jani was monitored around the clock for ten days by hospital staff and video cameras. The results of the test seemed to confirm Jani's claim that he did not eat or drink anything, and there were no drastic changes observed in his physiological condition. In the second test, from April 22 through May 6, 2010, Jani was observed by a team of thirty-five researchers from the Indian Defence Institute of Physiology and Allied Sciences, and other organizations.

The results were again pronounced as intriguing, with no deleterious effects observed in Jani's physical condition. So far, neither of these observational tests has been published in medical journals, and the studies have, of course, generated criticism. Skeptics have proposed that perhaps Jani escaped scrutiny of the hospital staff and video cameras through the assistance of his disciples, and that he did eat or drink something.[161] The hospital claims no, he was monitored continuously as they reported. In any case, if he did eat or drink surreptitiously, he would have had to eventually use the bathroom, and again the hospital reports that he didn't. In sum, with the evidence at hand it appears that Jani's claim corresponds to a known siddhi.

The second case is a doctoral-level chemist named Michael Werner, a managing director of a pharmaceutical research institute in Switzerland.[162] In his 2005 book, *Leben durch Lichtnahrung*, published in English in 2007 as *Life from Light*, he describes his interest in a twenty-one-day process developed by Australian spiritual teacher Jasmuheen, which supposedly allows one to transition from eating to not-eating. He tried the method, found it a relatively easy process, and now claims to have stopped eating solid food since January 1, 2001. In a ten-day observational test in October 2004, conducted in the intensive care ward of a hospital in Switzerland, Werner participated in a test similar to Prahlad Jani's. And, as in Jani's case, the results have yet to be published. Unlike Jani, Werner is a Western-trained scientist who is well aware of the standard skeptical arguments. And yet he is willing to participate in experiments to find out what is going on.

Perhaps the most curious aspect of the breatharian tests is the in-your-face nature of the claimed phenomenon and yet an almost complete lack of interest from the scientific community. If it is possible to live well without eating food, this ought to be easy to demonstrate, and if it held up, the scientific and social consequences would be astounding.

One explanation for the startling lack of interest is that most mainstream scientists and medical researchers regard this claim as so unlikely that they don't want to waste their time with it. Another is that those who studied the phenomenon may have actually discovered positive results, but they know how science reacts to "impossible" claims. So it's just safer to let positive studies quietly fade away.

A third interpretation is that the Jani and Werner studies actually found nothing out of the ordinary. In that case we might have expected both the Indian and the Swiss hospital teams to be happy to publish their negative findings, because that would only increase their perceived competence in the eyes of the mainstream. But that hasn't happened either.

There's a parallel here with psi studies. There is social pressure in the scientific community to publish results that conform to mainstream beliefs and expectations, and equally strong pressure to withhold results that might be perceived as strange or questionable. Critics are fond of claiming that if a robust psi effect was published in a prominent peer-reviewed journal, then other scientists would stampede to conduct replications, because surely wouldn't everyone love it if telepathy or clairvoyance turned out to be real?

This might sound reasonable, except that such stampedes are extremely rare. Exact replications of unexpected claims are critically important, but science—especially as it is practiced in academia—places more value on developing new ideas rather than on repeating old work, so there isn't much incentive. In addition, attempting to seriously repeat another scientist's claim will deflect time and energy from one's primary interests, and in any case for truly unexpected effects most scientists will simply assume that the replications aren't going to work anyway, so why bother?

Yoga, Psi, and Science

In considering what laboratory science has learned about the relationships between yoga and psi, a convenient way to classify the literature is in terms of Patanjali's eightfold path. The table on page 128, from transpersonal psychologist William Braud, shows the primary connections.[163] For the first two stages of the eightfold path, *yama* and *niyama* (the ethical and behavioral disciplines of yoga), virtually no psi research has been performed, so we don't know whether development of those factors influences psi performance.

For the next two stages, *asana* and *pranayama* (bodily postures and breath control), a small body of research has examined the influence of relaxation, hypnosis, and physiological states on psi performance.[164, 165] The literature suggests that these practices do improve psi performance, and probably for the same reason that they improve meditative practice—they reduce the mental "whirlings" that distract the mind.

For the fifth stage, *pratyahara* (sensory withdrawal), there is extensive psi research literature on telepathy in the dream state and in the "ganzfeld" (German for "whole field") condition.[166] This is the area with the strongest historical link between the *Yoga Sutras* and psi research, as these studies were actually designed with *pratyahara* in mind,[167, 168] but expressed in terms of physiological noise reduction, that is, as calming of the nervous system. Such a state was thought to possibly allow subtle psi "signals" that are always present to be perceived through the agitations of the nervous system and the distractions of the senses. The psi literature supports the notion that *pratyahara* improves psi performance.

For the last three stages, *dharana, dhyana,* and *samadhi* (stages of meditation), there is a modest body of research that focuses on whether various forms of meditation practice enhance psi performance.[169, 170] The results suggest that they do.

PSI Research Area	Yogic Practice
	Yama (restraints)
	Niyama (observances)
Relaxation	Asana (postures)
Hypnosis	Pranayama (breath control)

Physiological states

Dream telepathy   Pratyahara (sensory withdrawal)

Ganzfeld telepathy

Visualization in clairvoyance   Dharana (concentration)

Visualization in psychokinesis

Meditation   Dhyana (meditation)

Absorption   Samadhi (absorption)

Summary

Is it possible to use the tools of science to investigate the siddhis? Yes, to the extent that the phenomena are amenable to objective measurement. Some of the more extreme siddhis, like the ability not to eat or drink for indefinite periods of time, have been investigated in a few cases with intriguing outcomes. But the scientific taboo about taking these phenomena seriously limits the ability to conduct these studies at all, and so for the most part when it comes to the "big" siddhis, the jury is still out. This is not the case when the siddhi can be examined in the laboratory. Let's begin our survey of controlled laboratory tests with the first siddhi mentioned by Patanjali—precognition.

CHAPTER 9

Precognition

Yoga Sutra Pada III. Sutra 16: Knowledge of the past, present, and the future.

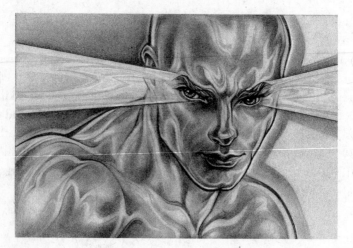

Precognition

The first siddhi described by Patanjali is the ability to simultaneously perceive the past, present, and future. Perceiving the present is not surprising; we call it awareness. Recalling the past is also not surprising; we call it memory.

While perceiving the present is not especially remarkable, explaining it is not so easy. Awareness is self-evident to everyone except for neuroscientists who are trying to explain how it is possible for the brain—a three-pound lump of tissue—to be aware of itself. This remains a major scientific mystery. It is almost as mysterious as the hard-core neuroscientists who have convinced themselves that their sense of awareness, and yours, is an illusion.[171] (An illusion to whom, they don't say.)

Perceiving the future, however, is a whole new ball game. Some philosophers think it is logically incoherent to gain information about the future, so for them precognition—perceiving the future—is literally impossible. Scientists, especially those with little knowledge of physics, tend to agree with the philosophers. But not all are so certain, as physicist Henry Margenau explained:

> Strangely, it does not seem possible to find the scientific laws or principles violated by the existence of [psi phenomena like precognition]. We can find contradictions between [their occurrence] and our culturally accepted view of reality—but not—as many of us have believed—between [their occurrence] and the scientific laws that have been so laboriously developed.[172]

Despite challenges to common sense, throughout history people have reported intuitive hunches, premonitions, and forebodings, some of which were later verified to be correct.[173] Some impressions that appear to be precognition are best understood through conventional means, as instances of coincidence, selective memory, forgotten expertise, implicit inference, confabulation, or fraud.[174] But are *all* cases of apparent foreknowledge accounted for by such explanations?

Attempting to answer this question with anecdotes will not get us very far; anecdotes carry little currency in science. It is well known that eyewitness testimony is too unreliable to provide credible data about controversial issues. But repeated personal experiences *do* provide the motivation to look seriously into these phenomena in the laboratory.

For some scientists and philosophers, precognition experiments reporting positive results do have a noticeable effect: They cause faces to turn red and sputtering noises to be issued by upset lips. For the general public, those very same studies are not nearly as exciting as hair-raising true tales of premonitions, nor are arguments based on statistical inference very persuasive. But the evidence they provide is far more credible because conventional explanations are strictly excluded.

Four classes of laboratory experiments have evolved to test if it is possible to gain information from the future under conditions that exclude inference, sensory clues, and all other ordinary explanations. The goal of these studies is to allow the investigator to state a clear hypothesis such that if precognition is present, then the experiment will produce one outcome, and if it is not present, then the experiment will produce a different outcome.

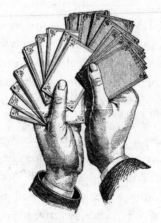

Forced-Choice Experiments

The first class of precognition experiments, known as "forced-choice" studies, was popularized by Joseph B. Rhine and his colleagues at Duke University starting in the 1930s.[175] In a typical experiment, a person might view five cards, each with a different symbol: a cross, wavy lines, a circle, a square, or a triangle. This set of symbols was used extensively in Rhine's early research. They are known as Zener cards, named after psychologist Karl Zener, who designed them.

In these tests, over a set of repeated trials, participants are asked to select one of the five cards that they think will be selected later by a random process. These tests use a metaphor of a target shooting game, where the goal over many repeated efforts is to aim at a target and hit it, so the words *hit*, *miss*, *target*, and *trial* are common jargon.

If a person's choice is correct, then this is counted as a hit, otherwise it is a miss. For a test with five possible targets, by pure chance we would expect the participants to select the correct target 20 percent of the time. If after many repeated trials the participants obtained hit rates higher than 20 percent, then it suggests that they used precognition to correctly anticipate the future choices, assuming that no clues were available about the identity of the upcoming cards. Simple statistical procedures are then used to judge whether the observed hit rate was significantly greater than expected by chance.

Targets in the early precognition studies typically included Zener cards or regular playing cards, and the random selection mechanism ranged from card shuffling to dice tossing. As electronics and computers became more commonly available, fully automated techniques were developed to select the targets using random methods based on quantum mechanical events (these are considered to be impossible to outguess, even in principle), and to automatically record the results of each trial.

Between 1935 and 1987, some 309 forced-choice precognition experiments were conducted by 62 investigators and published in 113 articles in peer-reviewed professional journals. More than fifty thousand people contributed nearly two million individual trials to these studies, and the time interval between the participants' choices and generation of the future targets ranged from a few milliseconds to a year.[176]

Meta-Analysis

To assess whether this collection of studies provided evidence for precognition, psychologists Charles Honorton and Diane Ferrari conducted a systematic, quantitative literature review called a *meta-analysis*. Meta-analysis is used extensively in the life sciences, from ecology to biology, psychology, and medicine. It uses strictly defined methods to combine data from many experiments, all of which were designed to study the same underlying phenomenon. This creates the statistical equivalent of a single, gigantic study.

The reason that meta-analysis has become popular is that living systems are so variable, and the effects of interest in an experiment are often so subtle, that it is difficult for any one experiment to provide persuasive evidence. In addition, credibility in science is strongly associated with whether a claimed effect can be successfully repeated by independent scientists. Meta-analysis allows us to see both whether a claimed effect is likely to exist, and whether it has been repeatedly observed by separate groups.

Among the 309 forced-choice experiments, the combined result showed a small but repeatable effect, with odds against chance of 10^{25} to one. That's ten million billion billion to one.[177] This means that the target was hit far too often for it to be considered a chance effect, suggesting that on average this group of people demonstrated a real skill—in this case, precognition.

Why isn't precognition accepted within mainstream science with experimental results of over ten million billion billion to one? One reason is that it's known that researchers tend to publish successful studies and withhold the rest, leading to a selective reporting dilemma known as the "file drawer problem." This problem can inflate the statistical assessment of a meta-analysis, and recognition of the problem has led to ways of estimating how many failed studies might remain buried somewhere in the file drawer, and also whether those hypothetical studies might be sufficient to reduce the known outcome to chance.

In this case, it was estimated that the hypothetical file drawer would require forty-six unpublished studies for *each* known experiment to reduce the outcome to chance. The rule of thumb for assessing whether the file-drawer effect is a plausible explanation is an estimated ratio of five to one unpublished to published studies. So in this case it is considered highly unlikely that the estimated number of unpublished studies could outweigh the known studies. Further analysis showed that twenty-three of the sixty-two investigators (37%) had reported successful studies, so the combined results were not due to just a couple of wildly successful, and thus possibly suspicious, investigators.

Another concern about a meta-analysis is that maybe the experiments that showed positive outcomes were just designed poorly, and conversely the studies with no evidence had excellent designs. If this were the case, then if we assessed the quality of the methods used in each study, and then compared those assessments to the actual study outcomes, we would expect to find a negative relationship (i.e., the better the design, the worse the results).

Among the forced-choice studies examined for this meta-analysis, 246 were described in sufficient detail to allow for a quality analysis. Rather than finding a negative relationship, a small *positive* relationship was found between study quality and effect size, so the results were not attributable to variations in experimental quality.

One other check that is often performed involves comparing the size of a measured effect in smaller versus larger studies. This is because if the effect examined in these experiments is genuine, then studies with more individual trials, or with more participants, should provide more confidence that the effect is indeed real.

Statistical aside: To see why, let's say we suspect that a coin is slightly biased. We think that when the coin is flipped, it will produce heads 51 percent of the time instead of 50 percent. If we flipped the coin 100 times, then on average we might indeed find an excess of 1 head. This 1 percent increase over chance confirms our expectation, but would a test with only 100 coin flips provide enough confidence that the coin is really biased?

It turns out that the answer is no. With just 100 flips, the odds against chance associated with observing 51 heads instead of 50 heads are only about 2 to 1. This is not very persuasive. So we do the experiment again, except this time we flip the coin 100,000 times. Again, when we add up the results we find the same 1 percent bias toward observing heads instead of tails, which in this case comes to a total excess of 1,000 heads. But now when we calculate the odds against chance of this 1 percent, we find that it is *7.8 billion* to 1. This provides very persuasive evidence that the coin is indeed biased. Why did the odds change so much? Because when you repeat an experiment many times, you gain progressively more confidence in the actual underlying effect.

This coin flip example is analogous to the small effects often obtained in forced-choice psi experiments. If the effect is genuine, then we should expect that studies with more trials should provide better evidence than smaller studies. That is, we would expect a positive relationship between study size and the statistical outcome of an experiment. This is what the forced-choice precognition meta-analysis found.

Is all this sufficient evidence to accept that precognition is real? From a hopelessly skeptical perspective, no, it isn't. Some scientists think that the whole idea of precognition is ridiculous, and some philosophers think precognition is *logically* impossible, so it cannot exist regardless of any evidence provided.

Thus, to demonstrate a persuasive supernormal effect, we need more than just evidence—we need *superevidence*. To work toward that goal, let's consider other types of precognition experiments to see if different approaches lead to the same conclusions. But before we go there, we need to take another short detour to examine the issue of "effect size," because it will come up again and again in our discussion.

Effect Size

It is sometimes imagined that the smaller an effect, the more likely it is due to a mistake rather than a real phenomenon. Who cares about things that are so small that you can hardly see or measure them? Maybe there are UFOs landing on the White House lawn on a daily basis, but if they're so small that even insects aren't paying any attention, why should we care? Well, the next time you get a cold virus, which is only about thirty billionths of a meter in diameter, and are in the midst of hacking your lungs out, it may be useful to revisit this question. When dealing with questions of "Is it real?," size definitely does *not* matter.

However, it is true that when dealing with weak effects and small-scale experiments, it may be difficult to detect what you're hoping to observe because, like trying to tune in a weak radio station, the signal one hopes to find might be obscured by noise. This is why the technique of meta-analysis was developed. It allows us to gain high confidence in small effects, providing of course that the effects are real. Meta-analysis doesn't allow you to magically create effects that don't exist.

The meaning of "effect size" varies according to what is being measured. In our coin flipping example, a 1 percent effect size refers to obtaining heads 51 percent of the time instead of 50 percent as expected by chance with a fair coin. Other experiments may involve different designs, say using four or five targets instead of a simple two-choice heads or tails. This makes the *meaning* of a 1 percent effect different across different studies. In meta-analysis this can be a problem because many different kinds of studies may be combined into one grand analysis. This may sound like meta-analysis tries to combine apples and oranges, but that is not the case if all those studies are interested in the same underlying phenomenon—for apples and oranges, the commonality might be a question posed about *fruit*.

Various formulas have been developed to provide a common

measure of "how big" an effect is, regardless of the specifics of the underlying experimental methods. The effect size for the forced-choice precognition studies is 0.02, where effect sizes typically range from about −1 to +1, and where 0 means the experiment produces no discernible effect. So an effect size of 0.02 is quite small. But the important question is what sort of confidence do we have that this small effect is actually not zero? That depends on the uncertainty of the effect size, which is what a statistical analysis provides.

One way to interpret the meaning of effect size is to consider how much one variable influences another. Say we were interested in the relationship between intelligence and popularity, or social support and health outcomes. The effect sizes for these two example relationships are 0.10 and 0.11, respectively.[178] To judge how much these effect sizes explain variations observed in popularity according to variations in intelligence, or how much social support influences health outcomes, a statistical analysis requires that we simply square the effect size.

Thus, in our example we get approximately $0.10 \times 0.10 = 0.01$, or one in a hundred, or 1 percent. This means that while the relationship between popularity and intelligence is quite *real*, the observed effect only *explains* a tiny fraction of the observed variation. The rest of the variations, the other 99 percent, are explained by many other factors (e.g., attractiveness, body type, gender, personality, education, etc.).

In some contexts, such as drug therapies, even extremely small effect sizes are taken very seriously because of possible adverse consequences. For example, the effect size relationship between tamoxifen, a drug used to treat breast cancer, and major vein blood clots is only 0.01. The explanatory power of this relationship is thus very weak, with fewer than 1 percent of people taking tamoxifen likely to experience this problem. But the downside risk is so serious that this contraindication figures into a risk-benefit analysis.

By comparison, as noted, the average effect size for the forced-choice precognition tests is 0.02. It's quite a small effect, but the statistical assessment shows that it is also quite real.

Comparing Psi and Non-Psi Effect Sizes

How do effect sizes in psi research compare to more conventional effects commonly studied in the social and behavioral sciences? The question is an interesting one because as we'll see, some psi experiments have produced effect sizes that are in complete alignment with the magnitude of effects commonly observed in conventional psychological phenomena. We know this through an article published in 2003 by psychologist F. D. Richard and colleagues in the journal *Review of General Psychology*.[179]

Richard's team reviewed one hundred years of social psychology studies, involving more than twenty-five thousand experiments and some eight million participants, creating the largest social psychology database ever assembled. Their analysis combined results of 322 meta-analyses of topics ranging from the study of aggression to gender roles, motivation, and social cognition. They found that the average effect size over all twenty-five thousand studies was 0.21. Squaring this figure to determine how much an effect size of this magnitude explains variations in relationships, we find that it explains about 4 percent, leaving 96 percent unexplained.

Coincidentally, the recent excitement in astrophysics over the discovery of dark matter and energy reached a similar conclusion. That is, if present cosmological models are correct, then the entire theoretical edifice for the origins and structure of the universe rests upon 4 percent of the detectable universe, leaving 96 percent completely unknown. Similarly, the scientific framework for biology firmly rests upon DNA, but as much as 96 percent of DNA has no known biological function, earning it the label "junk" DNA. Such fundamental unknowns will likely yield to future scientific advances, but the present state of ignorance should remind us to cultivate humility about what we think we understand. The fact is that the more science discovers about the nature of reality, the more we discover how little we actually understand.

Richard's article contained two other pertinent points that I've reproduced with a slight revision for reasons that will become clear:

> Psi research has grown over the past century. At the dawn of the 1900s, its experimental database consisted of a few studies. . . . More studies were conducted, and much was learned. Later, scholars began to question the evidentiary value of individual studies . . . and developed methods for synthesizing all of the research on a particular topic. . . . Now hundreds of research literatures have been meta-analyzed, and psi research can be quantitatively described.[179] (p. 339)
>
> The mean effect size yielded by a meta-analysis also requires judicious interpretation. Meta-analytic means . . . incorporate effects from a variety of conditions, settings, and research designs. Strong conclusions can be reached from research literatures that show homogeneous [i.e., similar] effect sizes. There, the mean is estimating a single effect. However, in research literatures that contain highly heterogeneous [i.e., different] findings, it would be naive to interpret the mean size of an effect as the magnitude of that effect under any particular set of conditions. . . . A psi effect may be larger under standard conditions than is the mean effect in the literature as a whole, the mean having been deflated by investigators' attempts to neutralize and reverse the usual finding.[179] (p. 340)

In the above quote, I substituted "psi research" for the article's original phrase "social psychology," and I used the phrase "a few studies" instead of the original article's "a single study." Otherwise exactly the same conclusions hold.

Free-Response Experiments

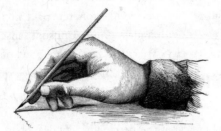

The forced-choice precognition experiments provide statistically impressive evidence for precognition, but the small effect size means that most of the time when people are selecting a future target, they're just guessing. This is discomforting to skeptics because it suggests that maybe those studies were hiding an undiscovered design flaw. And even if the tests were sound, forced-choice tasks are abstract, divorced from real-world concerns, boringly repetitive, and they encourage development of mental strategies to try to outguess the next target.

As a result, researchers began to develop "free-response" designs. These allowed test participants to freely report any impressions they might have gained about the future target, without restriction. The targets themselves were also revised, from simple colors and abstract shapes to photos of natural scenes, or to actual locations. Another important change was elimination of repetitive guessing strategies by conducting these experiments usually no more than once per day.

Consider one of the "precognitive remote perception" experiments conducted by Princeton University's Princeton Engineering Anomalies Research (PEAR) Laboratory. In this case the percipient (a person who attempts to perceive the future) and the agent (a person who would later travel to a randomly selected distant location) were separated by twenty-two hundred miles. In this example, forty-five minutes before the agent selected a site at random, the percipient described the following impression:

Rather strange yet persistent image of [agent] inside a large bowl—a hemispheric indentation in the ground of some smooth man-made materials like concrete or cement. No color. Possibly covered with a glass dome. Unusual sense of inside/ outside simultaneity. That's all. It's a large bowl. If it was full of soup [the agent] would be the size of a large dumpling![180] (p. 164)

With no idea about what the percipient had described, the agent was randomly assigned to visit the radio telescope at Kitt Peak, Arizona. If you did not know what a radio telescope looked like, the viewer's description is excellent—a hemispheric, smooth, man-made, large bowl. Keep in mind that this is just one example of hundreds of similar cases.

Many free-response precognition experiments have been reported by independent research teams, but the largest collection of relevant studies were produced by two sources. The first was part of a US government-supported, formerly classified program located first at SRI International in Menlo Park, California, from 1973 to 1988, and then at Science Applications International Corporation (SAIC), a large defense research and development company, from 1988 to 1995.[181] The second large body of studies was produced by the Princeton PEAR Laboratory from 1978 through the late 1990s.[182]

Analysis of 770 free-response tests conducted at SRI resulted in odds against chance of over 300 million to 1. Another 445 tests conducted at SAIC resulted in odds against chance of 1.6 million to 1.[181] At Princeton, a total of 653 sessions were conducted, resulting in odds against chance of 33 million to 1.[182] In each case the effect size reported by the two independent groups was virtually the same, about 0.20, which as we've seen is the same as the average effect size reported across tens of thousands of conventional social psychology experiments. This tells us that the magnitude of the free-response precognition tests is nothing special. It's what we should *expect* to find, on average, in a psychological test.

Similar effect sizes in the different free-response studies are also noteworthy because both teams were independently investigating the same phenomenon using similar methods, thus we should expect the effect sizes to be about the same. Notice also that the average effect size of these experiments was ten times larger than that obtained in the forced-choice studies. This confirmed the investigators' expectation that by using a method more closely aligned with how foreknowledge spontaneously occurs in the everyday world, and without the artificial constraints of forced-choice designs, more robust results should be obtained.

Presentiment Experiments

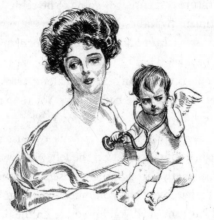

Encouraged by the success of free-response methods, investigators began to reason that because foreknowledge is commonly associated with visions, dreams, and other nonordinary states of awareness,[183] then perhaps *conscious* precognitive impressions are indistinct or distorted versions of information that is filtered through psychological biases. This speculation led to experiments designed to monitor bodily responses to future targets before those responses reached conscious awareness.

I began to conduct this type of experiment in the early 1990s, after reading about a few promising studies published decades before but apparently not followed up. I called these studies of *presentiment* rather than precognition to highlight the distinction between unconscious pre*feeling* as opposed to conscious pre*knowing*. I also decided to use experimental designs that were virtually identical to thousands of studies conducted within the conventional discipline of psychophysiology, anticipating that this might make the experimental paradigm more palatable to the mainstream, and because I could also employ commonly used methods of analysis.

In its simplest form, a presentiment experiment predicts that if the immediate future contains an emotional response, then that will cause more nervous system activity to occur *before* that response than it would if the future response was going to be calm. That is, the concept of presentiment hypothesizes that aspects of our future experience that we pay special attention to, like emotional upsets or startling events, "ripple backward" in time and can affect us now. A classical real-world example is when you're driving along a street, approaching an intersection, and you get a bad feeling. You're not sure why you have that feeling, so you slow the car down. You have a green light and there's no obvious reason to be cautious, but just as you reach the intersection a car from the street on the left, which was hidden by a building, careens wildly through the intersection. You suddenly realize with a shock that if you had continued driving at a normal speed that car would have smashed you broadside on the driver's side. The bad feeling in this case might have been caused by presentiment—a future moment of fright affecting you in the present.

In a typical presentiment experiment, the volunteer's nervous system is monitored continuously while he or she views a series of randomly selected stimuli. Measurements taken in these studies have included skin conductance (increased sweat), heart rate, variations in the size of the eye's pupil, brain electrical activity, and blood oxygenation in the brain.[184–190] The stimuli have included emotional versus calm photographs, stylized happy versus sad faces, audio tones versus silence, light flashes versus no flashes, and audio tones versus light flashes. To provide more concrete examples of presentiment experiments, let's examine a few that my research team and I have conducted.

Presentiment in Skin Conductance

To avoid awkward phrasing, we'll assume that the participant in our test is named Sally. To prepare Sally for this experiment, first we attach electrodes to two locations on her left palm. The electrodes record Sally's skin conductance level (SCL), which reflects the activation of her sympathetic nervous system. The term "conductance" refers to how easy it is for electrical current to flow; it's the opposite of electrical resistance. SCL is commonly used in lie detectors because if an individual tells a lie, and feels guilty, the person will sweat a little and that moisture will raise his or her skin conductance. Extremely small changes in SCL can be accurately measured, so SCL measurements are used extensively in experiments investigating human emotional responses to all sorts of stimuli (photographs, sounds, vibration, odors, etc.).[191]

The experiment uses a design whereby each target stimulus—in our example we'll use a photograph—is determined at random immediately before it is displayed. Sally is not familiar with any of the photos in the target pool; she's told only that the photos she'll see will range from very calm to very emotional.

When she's ready to begin, Sally clicks a mouse button and the computer screen she is sitting in front of remains blank for five seconds. Then the computer uses an electronic hardware circuit, a kind of very fast coin flipper called a "random number generator" (RNG), to randomly pick a color photo from a large pool of available pictures and then to immediately show it for three seconds. This is followed by a blank screen for ten seconds, providing a short cool-down period. Then a message appears on the screen instructing Sally to begin the next trial whenever she's ready.

This type of experiment might consist of thirty or forty such trials, each with a new randomly selected photo, and it takes around twenty minutes to complete. Sally is asked only to view the photo and to allow herself to feel any emotions associated with it. She is not to try to out-guess what she is about to see.

The stimulus photos consist of calming scenes, such as a landscape or a lamp, or emotional scenes with erotic or violent content. Photos used in various implementations of this experiment have come from professional stock photographs, web-based photo archives, and a picture set called the International Affective Picture System, the latter developed for the US National Institutes for Mental Health as a standardized set of photographs that are used worldwide in the study of human emotional responses.[192]

To analyze the results of the experiment, SCL data recorded during test sessions are averaged separately for all emotional and calm trials. These average curves are set to a common baseline value at the moment when the button is pressed to begin each trial, and then the prestimulus differences between the curves for the two target categories are calculated. Figure 2 shows the results of an experiment involving forty-seven participants who together contributed a total of 1,410 trials.[185]

The presentiment effect in this study is observed as the separation in the SCL signal from the moment that the trial begins (at −6 seconds in this study) to the moment that the photo is randomly selected and displayed (at 0 seconds). The difference between these two curves before the stimulus is shown may not look very impressive, but when it is evaluated statistically, it turns out that it is very unlikely to have occurred accidentally, with odds against chance of 2,500 to 1.

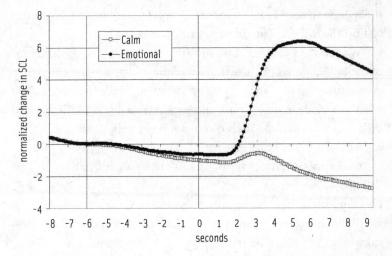

Figure 2. Average skin conductance across all calm and emotional trials. The button press to begin each trial occurred six seconds before the stimulus, a randomly selected picture appeared at 0 seconds, and the photo was displayed on a computer monitor for three seconds. Statistical analysis of the prestimulus curves from −6 to 0 seconds results in a difference associated with odds against chance of 2,500 to 1.

Presentiment in the Eye

In another study, we decided to record unconscious changes in each participant's left eye *before* they viewed randomly selected photos. We chose the eye as the measurement of interest because of cross-cultural superstitions about special forces attributed to the eye. From the power of "fascination" attributed to the evil eye, to the Hindu and Buddhist symbols for enlightenment, to the omniscient Eye of Providence on the US dollar bill, the eye is thought by some to emanate mysterious "energies" that are widely feared and revered.[193]

Sigmund Freud called fear of the evil eye "the most uncanny and universal" superstition, and there are innumerable legends of prophets or seers whose extraordinary gaze was said to divine the future. We wondered if these ancient superstitions—which are still vibrantly alive today, as witnessed by thousands of websites selling amulets to protect against the evil eye—might contain a grain of truth.

We knew of another class of experiments suggesting that some of the folklore might be worth reexamining. Meta-analyses of experiments studying the "sense of being stared at," under conditions that strictly exclude sensory cues and expectation biases, indicate that on average humans do indeed respond both consciously and unconsciously to another's unseen gaze.[194, 195]

Other meta-analyses testing mind-matter interactions with random physical systems, which we will examine in more detail later, also support the idea that highly focused intention, such as that associated with an intense gaze, appears to influence aspects of the physical world.[196, 197] Based on those experiments, combined with folkloric beliefs about the eye, we decided to investigate whether a "seer" could indeed see the future, and specifically whether we could detect such abilities in the human eye.

To do this, we considered another common belief about the eye, one that is no longer regarded as superstition. The poetic description of the eye as the "window to the soul" proposes that thoughts and feelings are reflected in the behavior of the eyes.[198] In psychophysiological terms, subjective states can indeed be inferred from pupil dilation, spontaneous blink rate, and eye movements.

For example, the size of the pupil is commonly used in the laboratory to study attention, cognitive processing load, emotional responses, anticipation, and the degree of balance between sympathetic and parasympathetic activation.[199, 200] The sympathetic portion of the autonomic nervous system, so-called because it is associated with "automatic" processes like breathing that don't require conscious control, is associated with nervous arousal; the parasympathetic portion is associated with relaxation. Eye gaze direction is monitored because it reflects the real-time allocation of attention,[201] mental imagery while imagining a scene,[202] and preferential processing in the left versus right brain hemisphere.[203] Moreover, the spontaneous rate of eye blinking increases with a rise in dopamine, a brain neurotransmitter associated with factors as diverse as fine motor coordination, insulin regulation, physical energy, and emotional response.[204]

Based on previous presentiment studies, the effect we were predicting to find would be most easily detected with increases in sympathetic nervous system activity. That would be associated with dilation of the pupil, so we predicted that we'd find larger pupils before emotional events than before calm events. We also speculated, based on differences in information processing in the brain hemispheres, that presentiment information might be processed more in the right brain hemisphere (in right-handed people) than in the left hemisphere. We further assumed that because eye movements reflect mental imagery, then people who showed significant presentiment effects in their pupil might also show correlations between their eye movements recorded *before* versus *while* viewing a stimulus photo.

We used a video eye-tracking system to monitor eye movement direction and to measure pupil diameter sixty times a second.[188] A computer controlled the experiment by coordinating the measurements obtained by the eye-tracking system with a second computer that was used to randomly select and display color photo images from the International Affective Picture System target set.

After we calibrated the eye-tracking apparatus to the participant's eye (let's call her Alice), the computer displayed a screen showing a uniform gray rectangle on a black background. When a "ready" message appeared on the screen, Alice clicked a mouse button and then the trial began. First the screen remained a uniform gray color for three seconds, then the computer used a random number generator to select a photo from the photo pool and display it for three seconds, and then the screen returned to a uniform gray for three more seconds. At this point a message appeared on the screen informing Alice that she could continue to the next trial whenever she was ready.

Because images in this study were selected at random from a collection of more than seven hundred photographs representing a very wide range of emotionality, most of the images that Alice viewed would have had emotionality ratings that were not especially emotional or calm, but somewhere in the middle.

The presentiment effect predicts that physiological measurements before a stimulus occurs will mimic the same measurements after the stimulus, thus to most easily detect this relationship we had to ensure that the poststimulus responses showed a strong calm versus emotional contrast. To do this we selected from the set of trials conducted by Alice and other participants only those photos with the 5 percent most emotional and 5 percent most calm images, where the emotionality of each photo was based on preestablished international standards.

Our study involved thirty-three volunteers. Together they contributed a total of 1,438 usable trials. Thirty-one subjects were right-handed and the remaining two were ambidextrous. This was important to track because we were interested in examining which hemisphere of the brain would respond more to presentiment, and this required that we use people with similar hand dominance. At the planned 5 percent level of emotional contrast in the target photos, the presentiment effect in pupil dilation was significantly positive as predicted, with odds against chance of 1,250 to 1 (see Figure 3). We also found significantly more spontaneous eye blinking before the emotional versus calm photos.

Five of the thirty-three participants showed independently significant presentiment results in their pupil dilation measurements. We examined their eye movements *before* the stimulus photo appeared, and we found a small but significant correlation between those eye movements and the eye movements recorded *while* they were viewing the photos. By comparison, we selected five other participants who did not show any evidence for presentiment, and in that group we found no correlation between their eye movements before versus while viewing the photos. This suggests that people who exhibit presentiment are not just responding to their future emotions, but also to visual information that is *specific* to those future targets.

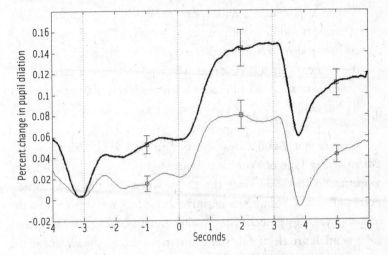

Figure 3. The top line shows the average proportional change in pupil dilation for the 5 percent most emotional targets over all 1,438 usable trials; the bottom line shows the same for the 5 percent calmest targets. Both lines are baseline adjusted to the average pupil dilation value recorded in each trial during the 167 milliseconds before the trial begins (just before second -3). Stimulus onset is at second 0 and stimulus offset at second +3. The error bars shown are plus and minus one standard error of the mean, and the curves are smoothed 500 milliseconds to help clarify the figure.

This experiment demonstrated that the autonomic nervous system as a whole, reflected in pupil and eye movements, unconsciously responds to future events. That is, it confirmed that there wasn't anything magically unique about skin conductance measures, as used in the initial presentiment effects.

Presentiment in Brain Activity

Some of our colleagues became intrigued by these experiments and they began to successfully repeat them,[187, 190] so we decided to expand our design to look at presentiment in the central nervous system—the brain. Our first attempt was based on a simple idea proposed in 1961 by British statistician Irving J. Good, who wrote:

A man is placed in a dark room, in which a light is flashed at random moments of time. . . . The man's EEG (electroencephalogram) is recorded on one track of a magnetic tape, and the flashes of light on another. The tape is then analyzed statistically to see if the EEG shows any tendency to forecast the flashes of light.[205]

We thought Good's idea was intriguing because "slow cortical potentials," a type of slow brain wave, have been used to study anticipation in the brain since the 1960s, when the first slow cortical potential, called "contingent negative variation," was reported by the psychophysiology pioneer Grey Walter and his colleagues. Slow cortical potentials are electrical oscillations measured on the surface of the scalp, where each oscillation may take a few seconds or more. This is in contrast to, say, the better-known "alpha rhythm" of the brain, which is about ten cycles per second. As an interesting historical sidelight, Grey Walter, who was not known for having an interest in psi, explicitly recommended that slow cortical potentials might prove to be useful for studying presentiment effects. It turns out that he was right (precognition?).

Shortly after Walter described the contingent negative variation, another slow cortical potential was identified and called the *Bereitschaftspotential*, or "readiness potential," which is associated with the anticipation of motor movements. Later, the contingent negative variation was found to consist of different components, and more recently other slow cortical potentials, generically called "stimulus-preceding negativity," have become a popular focus of study.

Based on these lines of research, physiological anticipation is now regarded in the neurosciences as a state in which brain areas required for specific cognitive operations become activated in advance of their use. For example, if you anticipate seeing something important, then the occipital region in the back of the brain, where visual input is processed, would become activated. Anticipation of emotions might activate the right frontal area, and so on.[206]

This brain-area specificity, combined with Good's idea, suggested a simple presentiment experiment we could conduct that involved brain activity. We predicted that we would find slow cortical potentials behaving differently just before a light flash than before a no-flash control. Based on previous presentiment studies involving electroencephalograph (EEG) measures,[207] we guessed that this effect would become most evident about one second before the stimulus. And because the anticipated stimulus in our design was simply a light flash, the main changes we expected to see would occur over the brain's visual processing region, the occipital lobe. To provide the simplest possible design, we took a single measurement over the occipital lobe.

Let's call our participant Susie. We prepped Susie with the appropriate electrodes and continuously recorded her brain activity throughout an experimental session. As she relaxed in a comfortable chair, she wore a pair of visual stimulator glasses that had three bright white light-emitting diodes (LEDs) mounted in these glasses in front of each eye. The glasses were controlled by a circuit that energized the LEDs on demand by a computer.

As in other presentiment experiments, Susie was asked to press a mouse button at will. That started a timer that waited four seconds, and then a random number generator circuit was accessed by the computer to decide whether to illuminate the six LEDs or to keep them unlit. After the stimulus, the timer waited another four seconds and then the computer sounded a short click tone to signal the end of the epoch.

At this point Susie could begin the next trial at will. She was asked to complete one hundred of these trials in one recording session. During the four-second period before the stimulus, the flash or no-flash decision was not yet determined, and in this way the protocol was double-blind. That is, neither Susie nor I, nor anyone else on the laboratory team, or even the computer itself, knew what the upcoming stimulus would be. So from an orthodox point of view, the stimulus type was not just unknown, but *unknowable*.

To check whether the hardware, software, analytical procedures, or the electromagnetic pulse produced by the stimulator glasses might have inadvertently introduced mistakes that mimicked a presentiment hypothesis, after all experimental data were collected, we collected another set of one thousand trials using a "sham brain" (we used a ripe grapefruit). We attached the same electrodes and visual stimulator glasses to the grapefruit "brain," and we ran ten sessions of one hundred trials each using the same procedures employed in the experiment, but with one addition: Instead of asking a human to press a button to initiate each epoch, a computer timer was used to generate a random intertrial period, and then it automatically started the next trial. Why a grapefruit for a sham brain? Because the size is about the same as a human skull, and because afterward we could enjoy a delicious snack.

The experiment consisted of a total of two thousand trials contributed by thirteen females and seven males. Because the brain processes visual information somewhat differently in men and women, we evaluated the data separately by gender. For the female participants, the presentiment hypothesis was supported with odds against chance of 140 to 1. Males did not show a significant difference. Figure 4 shows the average female brain response before, during, and after the stimulus, after smoothing the signal a bit for the sake of clarity. The control test with the grapefruit brain showed no differences.

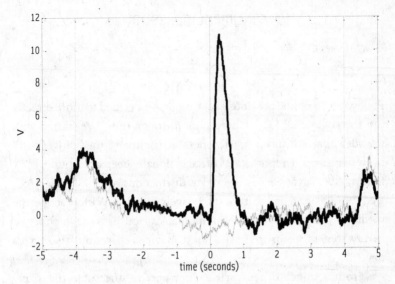

Figure 4. Brain electrical signals averaged across thirteen female participants, plus and minus five seconds from the moment of the stimulus (shown at time 0). After the light flash, there is a large rise in brain activity (bold line); after no flash (thin line), there is no change. When these same signals are traced backward in time, it can be seen that the brain was more activated one second before the light flash than before no light flash. The stimulus type (flash vs. no flash) was determined completely at random just before it occurred.

As usual in these studies, we explored whether this result might have been due to one or more unanticipated artifacts, including sensory and expectation cues, or procedural or movement artifacts. We found no evidence for such artifacts. Then, because I was kindly assisted in this study by Dutch psychologist Eva Lobach, who independently oversaw the recording of some of the participants, we examined the data to see whether the results we individually obtained might have been due to idiosyncratic differences in the way we interacted with the participants. We obtained the same results. Then we tested whether the results might have been due to one or two participants who produced unusually deviant outcomes. We found no evidence of that. In sum, this study indicated that the brain does indeed unconsciously anticipate future events, as Good had suggested.

Presentiment in Meditators

What does a clock do when it's hungry? It goes back four seconds.

Following up on the previous experiment, we decided to more directly test the yogic siddhi about perception through time. We started with the idea that advanced practitioners across many meditative traditions occasionally report states of exceptionally deep absorption.[208, 209] During such experiences, everyday distinctions such as subject/object, me/you, and past/future subjectively dissolve. With practice, the meditator may achieve a state of mental spaciousness in which his or her awareness seems to extend not just across space, but also across *time.*[210]

From a standard neuroscience perspective, the subjective experience of "timelessness" is explained as a brain-generated illusion.[211] But given the results of our other presentiment experiments, and successful replications of those studies reported by colleagues around the world, we felt that these experiences deserved a closer look. As we've already seen, Patanjali described that those who achieved stability in samyama and contemplated the nature of cause and effect would naturally begin to experience the ability to simultaneously perceive past, present, and future.[17, 18, 212, 213]

While many neuroscientists would not bother to test Patanjali's description, because they'd imagine that it couldn't possibly be true, it turns out that there is a class of temporal anomalies already described in the conventional literature that resembles the concept of timelessness. Terms like "precognition" and "presentiment" can even be found, albeit those terms are used in apologetic tones.

More often one finds euphemisms such as "exceptional situational awareness,"[214] referring to the performance of jet fighter pilots who respond faster in combat situations than they ought to be able to; "anticipatory systems,"[215] a phrase used to describe how organisms plan and carry out future behavior; and terms like "postdiction,"[216] "subjective antedating,"[217] "tape delay,"[218] and "referral backwards in time."[219] All these concepts are brain processes proposed to explain effects that look an awful lot like retrocausal (backward in time) effects. The underlying idea assumes that the brain has some sort of delay mechanism that fools us into consciously perceiving now what actually occurs at a later time.

It seems to me that the efforts used by neuroscientists to shoehorn retrocausal effects into standard neuroscience assumptions are reminiscent of the attempts of the medieval Scholastics to fit their epicycle models of the solar system into improved observations of the movement of the planets. That is, when astronomy was young, it was assumed that Earth was the center of the solar system and that heavenly bodies traveled in perfect circles (the "geocentric" model). As astronomical observations became more accurate, refinements to this idea became necessary. The Hellenistic astronomy of Ptolemy introduced the idea that planets moved according to multiple circles, known as deferents and epicycles. Later he added further adjustments called eccentrics and equants. All this reduced the elegance of the original geocentric models, and it made the process of calculating astronomical motions increasingly awkward. But it was also necessary, and the difficulties eventually led to more accurate sun-centered or heliocentric models of the solar system.

The point is that sometimes increasingly complex scenarios like "tape delays" in the brain are headed in the wrong direction, and it may be simpler to consider an alternative: What if the yogic perspective is actually correct? What if ordinary time perception is indeed an approximation of a deeper reality that resides beyond the everyday appearances of space and time? When that deeper reality is perceived from *outside* the confines of space-time, perhaps both past and future would be observed to influence the present.

Future influence on present awareness is what presentiment studies are designed to test, so my colleagues and I designed an experiment for sixteen subjects: eight advanced meditators, matched by age, gender, handedness, income, and ethnicity to eight nonmeditators.[220] We specifically recruited meditators with experience in practicing a *nondual* form of meditation because that style of meditation is associated with the experiential dissolution of dualities, including the dualism of "now" versus "then." Elements of nonduality can be found in many of the world's contemplative and philosophical traditions. These practices are best known in the West through the Dzogchen and Advaita forms of Zen meditation.[221]

Two simple stimuli were used in the experiment: a light flash and an audio tone. The light stimulus was a quarter-second flash provided by a pair of visual stimulator glasses; these produced a bright white flash about a centimeter in front of the eye. The audio tone was a moderately loud, short burst of noise provided over earbuds. The random decision to present an audio tone or light flash was made by a random number generator circuit, and another electronic circuit marked the electroencephalograph (EEG) record to precisely record the instant that the stimulus began. We measured each participant's brain waves with a thirty-two-channel EEG.

We fitted our participant, call her Lisa, with the electrodes, the visual stimulator glasses, and the earphones. She was told that the experiment would be conducted with her eyes closed, in two sessions of about fifteen minutes each, and with a five-minute break between the sessions. Each test session consisted of two tasks, and each task was repeated fifty times. The whole test session took about forty minutes to complete.

The first task asked Lisa to press a button at will. When she did this, three seconds passed, and then one of four possible stimuli was selected at random and immediately presented. The four possibilities were a light flash, an audio tone, a light flash and audio tone presented together, or no stimulus. These four possibilities were selected so the most likely stimulus type was no stimulus, and the other three were equally probable.

The second task began with Lisa pressing a button, then a random interval between two and six seconds was automatically generated. This was followed by a two-second prestimulus period, then by a randomly selected light flash, audio tone, or blank stimulus (each with equal probability). Two seconds later the next trial automatically began. In both tasks the stimuli we were interested in were the light flashes and audio tones. The other stimuli were used as distracters to reduce anticipatory or unconscious counting strategies, and to hide from Lisa which stimuli we were actually interested in.

The meditators in our study had an average of twenty-one years of a daily active practice; the nonmeditators had no active meditation practice, and most of them had never meditated at all. We predicted that the brain would show differences in electrical activity *before* unpredictable audio tones versus light flashes (because the brain processes these stimuli in different regions, thus creating different future brain states that might "ripple" backward in time).

The results of the experiment indicated that the nonmeditators showed no significant differences in brain activity before they received audio tones versus light flashes (see Figure 5). But in the meditator group, five of the thirty-two EEG electrodes showed statistically significant differences before receiving audio versus light stimuli (each electrode with odds against chance of 20 to 1) one second before the stimuli.

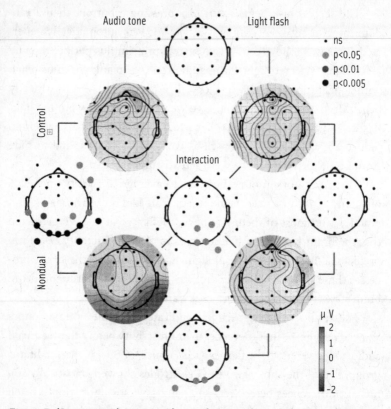

Figure 5. (Gray images) Average electrical potentials pooled across all trials in the meditation (labeled "nondual") and control groups, ranging from one second before the stimulus to stimulus onset, for all audio tone and light flash stimuli. Under the null hypothesis there should be no prestimulus electrical differences in the brain before the two stimulus types. (White images) Statistically significant comparisons between stimuli are shown as dots at each electrode site. All statistics are conservatively corrected for multiple comparisons.

In comparing brain responses between the meditator and the non-meditator brains, we found that before the audio tone, fifteen of the thirty-two EEG electrodes showed highly statistically significant differences distributed broadly over the cortex (with odds against chance in some of the electrodes at 200 to 1). This means that the meditators' brains behaved dramatically differently just before the audio tone, as compared to the nonmeditators' brains.

To help visualize the meditators' EEG activity before a light flash versus audio tone, we can examine the time-course of the EEG signal for one electrode (right superior centroparietal). Figure 6 shows the average EEG voltage for audio and light stimuli separately in the control and meditation groups, ranging from two seconds before the stimulus to one second after the stimulus. It shows that the meditators' brains behaved dramatically differently about 1.5 seconds before the stimuli were randomly presented, but there were no differences in the nonmeditators' brains.

This outcome supports the idea that these meditators were accessing future information in a way that is consistent with the first siddhi described by Patanjali.

But what's the big deal about 1.5 seconds? Remember that in the process of designing a controlled laboratory experiment we tend to end up with highly constrained, artificial versions of real-life experiences. The magnitude of the effects we see may not be impressive, but what we get in return is very high confidence that the effect of interest (in this case presentiment) is real. So responding to an event that will occur 1.5 seconds later in the laboratory may not help us avoid a disaster a month from now, but it does tell us that Patanjali wasn't spinning a fairy tale—*precognition is possible.*

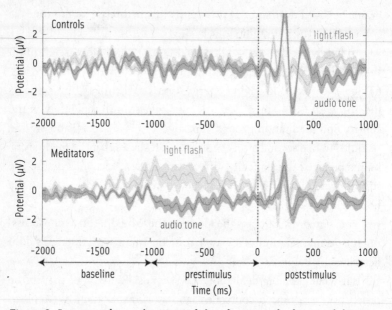

Figure 6. Average voltages (in microvolts) and one standard error of the mean envelopes, for light and audio stimuli, by group, at an electrode positioned over the right superior centroparietal region of the cortex. The signals are baseline adjusted from 2000 to 1000 milliseconds before the stimulus. Time 0 is the moment when the stimulus appeared. For ease of visualization these data were smoothed with a 10 Hz high pass filter.[220]

Presentiment Meta-Analysis

One presentiment experiment might provide interesting results, but what really captures scientific attention is when multiple, independent scientists report that they can successfully repeat an effect. When that happens, the effect is more likely to be real rather than an unnoticed artifact or a stupid mistake.

Is the presentiment effect repeatable? To find out, neuroscientist Julia Mossbridge of Northwestern University, psychologist Patrizio Tressoldi of the Università di Padova (in Italy), and statistician Jessica Utts of the University of California, Irvine, conducted a meta-analysis.[222] The presentiment studies they considered were published between 1978 and 2010, and they were required to have (a) analyses that were preplanned, (b) human physiological measurements recorded before randomly selected stimuli, and (c) clearly directional outcomes for expected effects both before and after the stimuli.

They found forty-nine published and unpublished presentiment experiments, of which twenty-six reported by seven laboratories fit their criteria. Five other laboratories reported similar studies, many of them reporting significant outcomes as well, but they did not fit the criteria for this particular meta-analysis. The twenty-six studies that they reviewed showed combined odds against chance ranging from 17 million to 370 billion to 1.

The odds figure of 17 million to 1 assumed that the presentiment effect varied randomly from one experiment to the next, which is the most conservative assumption. The odds figure of 370 billion to 1 assumed that the presentiment effect was constant across experiments, which is a more liberal assumption. The effect size in both cases was 0.21, by now a familiar effect size that appears repeatedly, on average, across all sorts of experiments involving human performance, including psi.

Mossbridge and her colleagues further found that higher-quality presentiment experiments resulted in larger effect sizes, which provides confidence that the reported results were genuine and not due to design mistakes. She also found that the number of unpublished file-drawer reports required to lower the overall level of significance to chance ranged from a conservative estimate of 87 studies to a more liberal estimate of 256 studies. Of those experiments that specifically explored whether the results might be due to anticipatory strategies or biases, no evidence of such biases was found.

So far, so good. The presentiment experiments are showing robust evidence for a repeatable, unconscious precognitive effect. But now we encounter a truly extraordinary piece of evidence that settles a common complaint about psi: If the claimed phenomenon is really true, then surely it would have been discovered long ago.

Well, perhaps it was, but no one was paying attention. And as it turns out, presentiment effects *have* been observed, completely unintentionally, in already published experiments conducted for other purposes.

Presentiment Everywhere

University of Amsterdam psychologist Dick Bierman, who had successfully conducted several presentiment experiments, reasoned that if this effect was really real, then it isn't magic—it ought to show up in other experiments too, even when the investigators weren't looking for it. To test this idea, he looked through the conventional psychophysiological literature to find experiments similar to those used in presentiment experiments, and he found three where data could be extracted from published graphs to explore whether there might be a presentiment effect.[169]

The first experiment was a study on the speed with which fear arises in animal-phobic versus nonphobic people; the second study was concerned with decision making, using a task known as the "Iowa gambling task"; the third study investigated the effect of emotional priming on the evaluation of Japanese characters. For all three studies, Bierman asked an assistant who was blinded to the purpose of the task to measure the skin conductance values in graphs appearing in the published reports.

Upon analysis of those values, in all three studies he found that before the stimulus occurred, skin conductance behaved as predicted by a presentiment effect, and when the data from all three studies were combined, it showed a result that was significantly in agreement with the presentiment concept. This confirmed his prediction that presentiment effects aren't magic, but are everywhere, *all the time*. You just have to look at existing data with new eyes to see it.

This is also completely consistent with the yogic lore claiming that our consciousness has access to vast amounts of information, but most of that information is suppressed by deep levels of the mind, so it rarely reaches conscious awareness. Through meditation training, one is said to gain better access to these deeper areas, and after extensive training one may gain full conscious access to this type of information.

If what Bierman found is really true, and presentiment effects are hiding in plain sight in data collected for other purposes, then it should be possible to repeat his finding with new data. Julia Mossbridge set out to test this idea. She and her colleagues investigated whether mainstream studies published after the year 2000, which is the year that Bierman published his analysis, would continue to show such evidence. She requested the raw data from fourteen researchers she identified, all of whom had published suitable experiments in mainstream physiology or psychology journals after 2000, and where each of those studies were investigating conventional hypotheses about human responses *after* stimuli. She was able to obtain the original data sets from two of those studies.

One study involved twenty-four participants with data recorded from the electrical signals associated with facial muscles (electromyography), skin conductance, heart rate, and skin temperature. All these measures were recorded continuously before, during, and after random presentation of four categories of photographs: neutral (e.g., a tree), pleasant-relaxing (a bunny), pleasant-arousing (an erotic couple), and unpleasant-arousing (a gruesome accident). Using highly conservative methods to examine these data, Mossbridge found no evidence for presentiment in the electromyography data, but she did find a positive effect in skin conductance and heart rate, and a significantly positive effect in skin temperature measurements (which is associated with flushing or blanching effects, which in turn is related to peripheral blood flow).

The second data set consisted of continuous skin conductance and brain-wave (EEG) data recorded before, during, and after the presentation of photos with pleasant low-arousing, pleasant high-arousing, unpleasant low-arousing, and unpleasant high-arousing imagery. Among the EEG electrodes with significant *post*stimulus effects, meaning those areas of the cortex that responded strongly to the images after seeing them, using her most conservative methods Mossbridge found significant presentiment differences in women participants (with odds against chance greater than 5,000 to 1), and similar but nonsignificant effects in the same electrodes in male subjects.

This mainstream study's original conclusion had been that women and men differ in how they responded *after* experiencing emotional events. Mossbridge found that this same conclusion held for how they responded *before* the emotional events. When she combined the pre-stimulus data across both genders, the odds against chance for a pre-sentiment effect were greater than 1,000 to 1.

Bierman's and Mossbridge's findings tell us that presentiment effects are ubiquitous. This means all of us are *unconsciously sensitive to future information all the time.* The first siddhi—awareness of past, present, and future—simply brings this awareness to consciousness.

All of this is consistent with the idea that the siddhis are refined expressions of everyone's potential. It suggests that if there's any one thing that prevents us from becoming siddhi superstars, it's our distracted minds and beliefs that act as filters to what we allow ourselves to perceive.

Implicit Behavior

The evidence for precognition doesn't end here. A whole new class of evidence has been developed since the turn of the twenty-first century.

The idea in these new studies is to time-reverse ordinary cause-and-effect sequences used in establishing well-known phenomena in the cognitive and social sciences. For example, in a conventional social psychology experiment a person might be asked to look at a pair of images presented on a computer screen. The images could be two of anything that can be more or less matched for similarity: two faces, two objects, or two abstract shapes.

The test participants' task is simple: select the one image from the pair that they prefer. Because the pairs of images used in these experiments were preassessed by independent judges to ensure that the two images in each pair were equally likable, then by chance you'd expect over multiple trials that each image would be picked about half the time.

To investigate a phenomenon known as the "mere exposure" effect,[223] a computer randomly selects one of the two images and repeatedly presents it subliminally (it flickers faster than individuals can consciously see) *before* the participants are asked to select which one they prefer. The test volunteers will have no conscious awareness of seeing the selected image, but when asked to select which one they like more, they will tend to select the image that they were exposed to subliminally. This experiment in the mere exposure effect demonstrates that we tend to like what we are familiar with, even when the familiarity is due to unconscious exposure before making a decision.

In the time-reversed twist to this experiment, the participant is *first* asked to select one of a pair of images, and then *after* the selection the computer randomly selects one of the two images and repeatedly presents it subliminally. This time-reversed design predicts that experiencing the image *in the future* will "leak backward" in time and bias the subject's *present* decision.

In a series of nine such experiments, all involving time reversal of conventional experiments, Cornell University psychologist Daryl Bem reported statistically significant evidence in eight of the nine experiments, which overall involved more than a thousand participants, mostly college students. His studies were published in early 2011 in the high-profile *Journal of Personality and Social Psychology*, with the title "Feeling the Future: Experimental Evidence for Anomalous Retroactive Influences on Cognition and Affect."[224] Across all nine experiments, the average effect size was 0.22, and the combined odds against chance were 73 billion to 1.[225]

Clash of the Paradigms

Besides providing a new form of evidence for retrocausal effects, Bem's paper serves as an excellent case study to show how normally calm, rational scientists and science journalists respond when they encounter unexpected results. In brief, they go berserk.

Before Bem's paper was even published, an editorial in the *New York Times*, published on January 5, 2011, was already whipping scientists into a frenzy. With the title, "Journal's Paper on ESP Expected to Prompt Outrage," science writer Benedict Carey could barely conceal his disdain:

> The decision may delight believers in so-called paranormal events, but it is already mortifying scientists. Advance copies of the paper, to be published this year in *The Journal of Personality and Social Psychology*, have circulated widely among psychological researchers in recent weeks and have generated a mixture of amusement and scorn. Some scientists say the report deserves to be published, in the name of open inquiry; others insist that its acceptance only accentuates fundamental flaws in the evaluation and peer review of research in the social sciences.
>
> "It's craziness, pure craziness. I can't believe a major journal is allowing this work in," Ray Hyman, an emeritus professor of psychology at the University of Oregon and longtime critic of ESP research, said. "I think it's just an embarrassment for the entire field."
>
> The editor of the journal, Charles Judd, a psychologist at the University of Colorado, said the paper went through the journal's regular review process. "Four reviewers made comments on the manuscript," he said, "and these are very trusted people." All four decided that the paper met the journal's editorial standards, Dr. Judd added, even though "there was no mechanism by which we could understand the results."

But many experts say that is precisely the problem. Claims that defy almost every law of science are by definition extraordinary and thus require extraordinary evidence. Neglecting to take this into account—as conventional social science analyses do—makes many findings look far more significant than they really are, these experts say.

Besides the bluster of asserting that a peer-reviewed scientific study accepted in a prominent journal was "pure craziness," it's unfortunately common to read about experts who go ballistic when learning about effects that supposedly "defy almost every law of science." In the same news article, cognitive scientist Douglas Hofstadter of Indiana University protested that, "if any of [Bem's] claims were true, then all of the bases underlying contemporary science would be toppled, and we would have to rethink everything about the nature of the universe."

Such alarming statements imply that scientific laws are carved in stone like the Ten Commandments, and thus they are impossible to violate, or at least they may be desecrated at risk of annoying Moses. In fact, all scientific laws are just regularities that are true on average in limited contexts. And in any case the "laws" that are supposedly violated are never specified for the simple reason that *there are no such violations*. Declarations like Hofstadter's are based on anxiety, not by sitting down calmly before the facts.

But the mere idea of precognition remains so upsetting to some scientists that it becomes easier for them to believe that basic scientific methods have suddenly and mysteriously soured, rather than to imagine that the offending claim might be true.

This is not an unreasonable first reaction, because methodological improvements are always possible. But it's actually a classic catch-22: To avoid facing the possibility that the "laws of science" are wrong, some time-honored techniques used in thousands of previously published experiments *must* be wrong. But here's the rub: Those very same, now presumably wrong, techniques were used to establish the precious laws of science in the first place!

In sum, we are required both to accept and to reject the same techniques.

This catch-22 is not new. In the 1930s, when J. B. Rhine's ESP card tests were showing remarkable success, critics insisted that the mathematical methods he was using must be flawed. They just *had* to be wrong. The debate persisted until the criticisms were conclusively rejected by the president of the Institute of Mathematical Statistics, who at the time was Burton Camp of Wesleyan University. Camp finally released a statement to the press, which was reprinted in the first volume of the *Journal of Parapsychology*. It read:

> Dr. Rhine's investigations have two aspects: experimental and statistical. On the experimental side mathematicians, of course, have nothing to say. On the statistical side, however, recent mathematical work has established the fact that, assuming that the experiments have been properly performed, the statistical analysis is essentially valid. If the Rhine investigation is to be fairly attacked, it must be on other than mathematical grounds.[226]

A modern example of this "something must be wrong" argument appeared in an editorial about Bem's study in the premier scientific journal *Science*. Entitled "ESP Paper Rekindles Discussion About Statistics," journalist Greg Miller reported that:

> "The real lesson to be learned from this is not that ESP exists, it's that the methods we're using aren't protecting us against spurious results," says David Krantz, a statistician at Columbia University.[227]

Another example is an article by journalist Bob Holmes in the magazine *New Scientist*, with the title "ESP Evidence Airs Science's Dirty Laundry."[228] The dirty laundry is identified in a quote from a statistician at Duke University: "An awful lot of what's published out there is wrong." Holmes then continues,

> Despite widespread scepticism from mainstream scientists, studies of precognition and other forms of extrasensory perception crop up time and again. In the 1940s it was card-guessing, in the 1980s the ability to influence random-number generators, and in the last decade so-called "presentiment"—in which volunteers showed changes in skin conductance just before they saw disturbing images. In every case, however, independent researchers failed to repeat the initial results, eventually concluding that they were the result of procedural flaws or coincidence.

As we've learned from our review of presentiment experiments earlier in this chapter, Holmes's opinion is spectacularly, stunningly wrong. He's also wrong about the other classes of psi experiments, demonstrating the amazing capacity to ignore what we don't want to see.

In another example, an article entitled "Fearing the Future of Empirical Psychology" was published in the *Review of General Psychology*. Psychologists Etienne LeBel and Kurt Peters squarely identified the impending problem:

> By using accepted standards for experimental, analytic, and data reporting practices, yet arriving at a fantastic conclusion, Bem has put empirical psychologists in a difficult position: forced to consider either revising beliefs about the fundamental nature of time and causality or revising beliefs about the soundness of [modal research practice].[229] (p. 371)

Bayesian Methods

In yet another critique, entitled "Why Psychologists Must Change the Way They Analyze Their Data: The Case of Psi," psychologist Jan Wagenmakers and his colleagues from the University of Amsterdam argued that a more appropriate statistical technique for analyzing this type of controversial data was to use Bayesian techniques, named after the eighteenth-century mathematician and theologian Thomas Bayes.[230] This method is useful because it objectively specifies how an investigator's previous beliefs ought to change when confronted with new data.

The method requires that the analyst specify two types of beliefs—one about how likely the "null" or chance hypothesis is to be true (statistical jargon calls this null hypothesis "H0"), and the other about how large the effect size would be if the alternative hypothesis is true (called "H1"). H1 in this case is the hypothesis that people *can* receive information from the future, and H0 is the hypothesis that they *can't*.

The process begins by specifying one's belief that people *cannot* receive information from the future (i.e., H0). Wagenmakers set these odds at a whopping 1,000,000,000,000,000,000,000 to 1, or a thousand billion billion to 1, reflecting his conviction that precognition is impossible.

The next step was to specify his belief about how effect sizes over many experiments would look if precognition were in fact true (i.e., the alternative hypothesis, or H1).

Specifying H1 is concerned with the range and distribution of effect sizes that one would expect to see after conducting many studies, rather than just an estimate of the effect size one would expect to see in a single study. The *shape* of the expected distribution of effect sizes is the critical issue, because that shape represents what one believes about the effect being studied. Is the expected effect assumed to be tiny and rare, or huge and common, or somewhere in between?

The outcome of this type of analysis is expressed in terms of a "Bayes factor," which is the odds of the alternative hypothesis (H1) compared to the null hypothesis (H0) *after* being presented with new experimental data.

Using this method, Wagenmakers evaluated each of Bem's nine experiments separately. His gigantic odds in favor of the null hypothesis, combined with his choice of the distribution for the alternative hypothesis, eliminated the possibility that *any* new data could influence his opinion in favor of precognition. So not surprisingly he concluded that Bem's study did not provide evidence for precognition after all.

Wagenmakers's paper was immediately published and embraced with a sigh of relief by the orthodoxy as a safe reason to ignore Bem's results. But was it valid?

Bem published a reply with coauthors Jessica Utts and Wesley Johnson, both professors of statistics at the University of California, Irvine.[225] In particular, Johnson was codeveloper of the statistical method used by Wagenmakers, and as such he was uniquely competent to judge if it was properly used. In their opening assessment, Bem and his colleagues calmly noted that "it requires careful thought to apply Bayesian methods correctly, and we believe that Wagenmakers et al. . . . have not done so" (p. 716).

It turns out that not only did Wagenmakers select unreasonable odds of a thousand billion billion to one in favor of the null hypothesis, he also selected a wildly unrealistic distribution for effect sizes that one should expect for a precognition experiment. In brief, Wagenmakers assumed that the results of a typical precognition study ought to include effects that were so huge that if that's how precognition really behaves, there wouldn't be any controversy over the existence of the phenomena. In other words, precognition according to Wagenmakers should be *both* a priori impossible *and* self-evidently obvious when studied in experiments.

In contrast to Wagenmakers's approach, rather than relying on personal beliefs to establish odds for H0 and H1, Bem, Utts, and Johnson selected values based on previously published experimental evidence for precognition. They also considered Bem's set of nine studies as a group rather than examining each one separately.

They found that the Bayes factor in favor of genuine precognition in Bem's experiments was conservatively 13,669 to 1. This means that if your prior belief *against* precognition is as high as 100 million to 1, then after being presented with Bem's data your belief ought to shift *toward* support for precognition, assuming that you were able to sit still long enough to behave rationally.

Bem, Utts, and Johnson ended their article by reconsidering Wagenmakers's question: Should psychologists change how they analyze data? They concluded that the answer was no, everything is just fine. But they did caution that any analysis must be conducted properly:

> This debate is an excellent illustration of how science works. Different individuals working on the same scientific problem come to different conclusions based on their own assumptions and models—which Bayesian methods make explicit. Such disagreements persist until there is sufficient information available to convince the broader scientific community where the truth lies. . . . Ironically, Wagenmaker et al.'s (2011) critique itself provides an illuminating example of how hidden flaws or artifacts can lurk "in the weeds" of an unfamiliar statistical analysis—albeit here in the service of defending the null hypothesis.[225] (p. 718)

Much more can be said about the statistics used to analyze psi experiments, but to fully appreciate those arguments would take us far beyond the scope of this book. The bottom line is this: The trembling in academic journals over how science must be falling apart because of positive evidence for psi is a desperate attempt to maintain a stable worldview where psi can't exist. But when correctly applied, scientific methods are exceptionally powerful and for the most part they are perfectly sound. The reality of psi does indeed challenge some scientific assumptions, but it does not mean we need to radically change everything we know.

At least not yet.

Bem's innovative approach is relatively new, and as such the jury is not yet in on whether the effect will be easily repeatable by others. As I was writing this chapter, several replication attempts have been reported. Some of those studies were successful; others failed to repeat the effect. Nineteen replications based on one of Bem's designs were meta-analyzed in a paper by Jeff Galak of Carnegie Mellon University and his colleagues.[231] Galak's review was entitled "Failures to Replicate Psi" in spite of the fact that only fifteen of the nineteen replications actually employed methods similar to those used by Bem. When those fifteen studies were considered as a separate group, they provided a significant, positive replication. The other four experiments were conducted online, which simplifies recruitment of participants but at the price of introducing many uncontrolled variables (which is why Bem did not conduct his experiments that way). Galak's paper further trumpets that their own attempted replications, seven in all, included 3,289 participants. This sounds impressive until you learn that over 80 percent of those people participated online. The devil is often in the details, and sometimes the details within articles reporting failures to replicate are not quite as negative as they are advertised.

Animal Presentiments

Similar to stories about precognition and presentiment in humans, there is a long history of animals reacting prior to major natural disasters, such as tsunamis and earthquakes.[232] Explanations commonly offered for such observations include animal sensitivities to geomagnetic, electromagnetic, and atmospheric disruptions just before such events. Another possibility is that, like humans, animals can sense the future.

Intrigued by the compounding evidence for human presentiment, researchers have begun to expand this line of research into animal behavior. This category of experimentation is relatively new, but three experiments are already providing intriguing reasons to believe that animals can indeed perceive the future. The studies involved earthworms, Bengalese finches, and Zebra finches.

In the first study, for his master's thesis in electrical engineering, Chester Wildey investigated whether earthworms would show a presentiment effect by using mechanical vibration to create the worm's equivalent of an emotional stimulus, and no vibration as a "calm," unemotional control.[233] His experimental results were consistent with outcomes reported in human presentiment experiments; that is, more activity prior to the stimulating vibration than before no-vibration. He also found that the more trials he collected, the more his data agreed with the presentiment hypothesis, which is what one would expect if the "signal" was a genuine one.

In the second study, Fernando Alvarez of the Estación Biológica de Doñana in Seville, Spain, placed forty-seven Bengalese finches (*Lonchura striata*) into a cage, one at a time.[234] After allowing the birds to become acclimated to the cage for fifteen minutes, a random number generator selected a random time to display a fifteen-second video clip on a video screen next to the bird cage. The video showed a horseshoe whip snake, *Coluber hippocrepis*, apparently crawling toward the birds. When Bengalese finches see this type of snake, they display distinctive alarm movements (that's ornithology jargon for "they freak out"). As a control test, Alvarez used the exact same procedure but no video clip was shown, and for a second type of control the birds' alarm behavior was measured ten minutes before the initial acclimation period.

The birds were continuously filmed during the experiment, and the frequency of alarm behavior was counted from 0 to 3, 3 to 6, and 6 to 9 seconds before the snake image appeared. The same procedure was followed for the control trials. To avoid being influenced by the condition, these counts were performed blinded to whether a given video clip occurred just before a snake appeared or no snake appeared.

The results showed that the birds reacted to the snake video clip up to nine seconds before it was shown, with the frequency of the alarm display during that period being significantly greater than observed in the first type of control, with odds against chance of 5,393 to 1. Based on the second type of control, the odds were even stronger: 280,000 to 1. By contrast, there was no difference in counts between the two types of controls.

In a third study with similar aims, Alvarez successfully replicated the Bengalese finch study using adult female Zebra finches (*Taeniopygia guttata*), using a startle stimulus (the sound of a gunshot) instead of a snake video.[235]

Summary

The accumulated evidence is clear: Precognition exists. In 2011, I presented some of the evidence discussed in this chapter at a physics symposium on quantum retrocausation. This was part of the Western Regional meeting of the American Association for the Advancement of Science, hosted that year by the University of San Diego.[236] The evidence for precognition was relevant to this symposium because retrocausation—a reversal of the usual cause-and-effect sequence— is entirely compatible with the equations of both classical and quantum physics. Physicists readily accept time reversal at the elementary particle level, but precognition in humans suggests that time-reversal phenomena also occur in the macroscopic, everyday world. As such, evidence for precognition plays a key role in physical theories that are attempting to model the fundamental nature of time, as well as understanding the transitions between the physics of the microworld and the macroworld.

The technical papers from the 2011 meeting, and for a similar symposium in 2006 on the "frontiers of time," were published in two books by the American Institutes of Physics,[236, 237] a leading publisher in the physical sciences.

Beyond the abstruse world of theoretical physics, throughout history ordinary people have reported hunches, premonitions, and foreknowledge about future events that were later verified to be accurate. Conventional explanations like coincidence and selective memory can account for many of these anecdotes. But for over seventy-five years, laboratory studies have investigated whether some of those experiences may be based on genuine time-reversed or retrocausal effects. As of 2012, the accumulated experimental database includes hundreds of laboratory studies reported from researchers in the United States, Italy, Spain, Holland, Austria, Sweden, England, Scotland, Iran, Japan, and Australia.[236]

Does this mean that people ought to be able to foresee every future disaster, or break the banks of the casinos or the stock market? No, because the effect sizes in these experiments are rather small. But as we'll see later, precognition can be used for practical applications. It also indicates that most humans do have at least one of the siddhis that yoga claims to be able to develop.

What else was Patanjali correct about? Can you read my mind?

CHAPTER 10

Telepathy

There are many books on how to win friends and influence people, but surprisingly few on how to make enemies and alienate people. Here is a suggestion to fill the gap. Walk into a group of scientists and announce that you believe in parapsychology.

—*Roger Walsh*

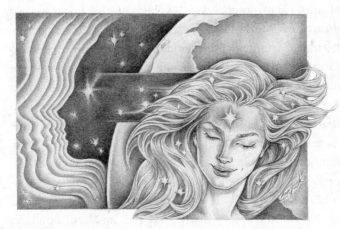

In the *Yoga Sutras*, *Vibhuti Pada* III.19–20 describes siddhis suggesting that it is possible to gain knowledge of others' minds. Today we would call this ability *telepathy*, a mind-to-mind connection. Like other psychic phenomena, reports of telepathic communications can be found across all cultures, and these experiences were just as common centuries ago as they are today.

Samuel Clemens, who used the celebrated pen name Mark Twain and was the author of such nineteenth-century classics as *Tom Sawyer* and *Adventures of Huckleberry Finn*, had many telepathic experiences. He dubbed them "mental telegraphy" because the telegraph was the fanciest long-distance communication technology in his day. Twain was concerned about his reputation as a serious author if he reported his experiences, so for years he kept quietly adding his experiences to an unpublished manuscript. Finally, after British scientists began to show serious interest in this topic in 1882 with the formation of the Society for Psychical Research, Twain decided to publish an article in *Harper's New Monthly Magazine* in 1891. It began:

> Note to the Editor.—By glancing over the enclosed bundle of rusty old manuscript, you will perceive that I once made a great discovery: the discovery that certain sorts of thing which, from the beginning of the world, had always been regarded as merely "curious coincidences"—that is to say, accidents—were no more accidental than is the sending and receiving of a telegram an accident. I made this discovery sixteen or seventeen years ago, and gave it a name—"Mental Telegraphy." It is the same thing around the outer edges of which the Psychical Society of England began to group (and play with) four or five years ago, and which they named "Telepathy."
>
> Within the last two or three years they have penetrated toward the heart of the matter, however, and have found out that mind can act upon mind in a quite detailed and elaborate way over vast stretches of land and water. And they have succeeded in doing, by their great credit and influence, what I could never have done—they have convinced the world that mental telegraphy is not a jest, but a fact, and that it is a thing not rare, but exceedingly common. They have done our age a service—and a very great service, I think.[238]

Twain may have overestimated the scientific community's reaction to evidence for telepathy, but he was right about the general public's interest. Today his stories about telepathy would be wildly popular and form the basis of a TV series.

Telepathy Tests

How do we go about testing whether an impression of telepathy is a coincidence, a hallucination, a psychiatric problem, a fabrication, or genuine? We'll use an example of two friends, Gail and Tom.

Gail tells you that she thinks she's in telepathic contact with Tom. She seems to know what he's thinking and vice versa, not literally with words but with intentions. She provides examples of spontaneous episodes that seem credible, and you know her well enough to accept that she's not making up these stories. You decide to test her ability.

You begin by asking Gail to think of any number, at random, from 1 to 10, then to multiply that number by 9. If the resulting number is two digits, then Gail should add the digits together, and then subtract 5. (You should try this too, to see what happens.)

Now you ask her to determine which letter in the alphabet corresponds to the number she ended up with (example: 1 = A, 2 = B, 3 = C, etc.).

Now ask her to think of a *country* that starts with that letter and to remember the last letter of the name of that country. Then ask her to think of the name of an *animal* that starts with that letter, and to remember the last letter in the name of that animal. Finally, ask her to think of the name of a *fruit* that starts with that letter.

Now ask Gail, are you thinking of a kangaroo in Denmark eating an orange?

If she is (and if you were), then you've learned the first lesson in how *not* to conduct a telepathy experiment. This trick works with the majority of native English speakers because we share common knowledge about the frequency of words and concepts, and this allows you to be led down the primrose path to ensure that you select the most common choices for those words. Magicians use similar tricks to force you to select a specific item that you think you're choosing freely, but actually you're just following well-known biases.

So let's look at another design for a telepathy experiment. First you have Gail and Tom sit back to back. You ask Tom to think of anything that comes to mind, and then you ask Gail to report what he's thinking. If you do this a few times, you may be amazed to find that occasionally Gail gets it exactly right. But maybe they've been passing clues through body positions or innocuous sounds. Or maybe they've decided to play a trick on you by secretly setting up a series of mental targets in advance.

So you separate them into different rooms and satisfy yourself that they can't communicate in any conventional way. Not with sounds, vibrations, odors, or cell phones, or even via a confederate who might be persuaded to secretly pass messages between them. Now you try the experiment again, asking Tom to think of something at random, and seeing if Gail gets it. Sometimes she does, and with wildly good accuracy. Still, something doesn't feel right. Surely telepathy isn't that easy. If it was, it wouldn't be considered controversial.

You decide that maybe because Gail and Tom know each other so well that what looks like amazing telepathic hits is actually due to shared knowledge. That is, if they both went sailing the day of the test, then it is likely that water sports would be on both of their minds, so Tom might select a water-sport-related item as his telepathic target. But so would Gail, because people aren't good at selecting items at random. Here's where the combination of common knowledge and recent memory can easily bias the results to make it appear that Gail was telepathic.

To get around this, you devise a method where you select one target photograph out of a large pool of photos with a broad range of content. To make that selection without introducing your own nonrandom decision biases, you toss dice, or shuffle cards, or use a computer-based method to choose the target. But now you wonder how are you going to judge how good the match is between what Gail says and what Tom's target was, without introducing yet more biases? If you select a photo with a red balloon, and Tom doesn't say "balloon" but he does report the color pink, is that good enough to count as telepathy?

So you make it easier to judge a hit or miss by selecting four photos, each as different from one another as possible, and then you randomly select one of those photos as the target to give to Tom. Now you can judge Gail's accuracy after Tom finishes mentally "sending" the target by showing Gail all four photos and asking her to select the one that best matches her impressions of what Tom was sending.

To avoid accidentally giving Gail a clue about which one of the four targets was the actual one, you decide to ask someone else to select the target photo and give it to Tom. Then, when you're with Gail and evaluating the test session, you have no idea which of the four photos is the target, and when you hand Gail the four targets to evaluate, you use fresh copies so that Gail never even sees the photo that Tom handled. Now Gail selects one of the four targets, and she either gets it right or not.

Okay, so now you conduct the test session using this design, and at the end Gail selects the correct target, and so you have proof of telepathy, right? Well, not quite.

Let's say that Gail's impression was about a dog, the target photo was a picture of an elephant, and the other three decoy targets were grass, a tree, and a bird. Gail selected the elephant because it was the only animal with four legs among the four targets. While this would count as a direct hit, it isn't a very impressive hit because she didn't actually say the target was an elephant.

Maybe she was having a bad moment. You run the test again. Again she gets a hit, but again it wasn't an exact match. So you run dozens of trials. Some are hits and some are misses. If Gail was not telepathic, then she should get the right answer purely by chance on average about one in four guesses, or 25 percent of the time. Barring telepathy, if the targets are really selected at random, there is absolutely nothing she can do to amplify this hit rate.

Now you decide to expand your test to include many different pairs of people. You gather data from dozens, then hundreds, then thousands of sessions because you want to see whether telepathy is true for people in general, rather than just for Gail and Tom. In the process of running these tests, you develop even more sophisticated controls to ensure that the participants can't cheat or introduce biases, you add other methods to prevent yourself or your assistants from cheating or introducing biases, you devise fully automated techniques to record the data properly, and you use statistical methods that are simple but appropriate to evaluate the data.

After running several thousand trials, you observe that the telepathic "receivers" are on average correctly selecting the randomly chosen target about one in three times rather than the chance-expected one in four. It doesn't seem all that impressive. But you calculate the odds against chance to see how unusual it is to get 33 percent when you'd expected to get 25 percent by chance, given the number of trials you've run. The outcome makes your head spin.

The above description is a brief recapitulation of the evolution of telepathy tests from the 1880s to today. A method designed in the 1970s, called the *ganzfeld* test, is the most recent iteration of our Gail-Tom test scenario. This design has become a standard technique used to test for telepathy. And it is directly relevant to our interest in the siddhis because the ganzfeld design was explictly developed to test whether telepathy would be easier to detect when sensory noise was reduced. This idea in turn was based on the yogic lore that withdrawal of the senses would assist the yogin to become more aware of subtle inner impressions, including telepathic experiences.

Ganzfeld

Ganzfeld is a German word meaning "whole field." It's a mild form of unpatterned sensory stimulation originally developed by gestalt psychologists to study the nature of perception and visual imagery.[239] In a ganzfeld experiment, the "receiver," Gail in our example, is asked to relax in a comfortable, reclining chair. The experimenter places halved Ping-Pong balls over her eyes and gives her headphones to wear that play pink noise, a whooshing sound like a deep-throated waterfall. Then the experimenter shines a red light on Gail's face, and she is asked to keep her eyes gently open under the Ping-Pong balls. All she'll see is a soft red glow everywhere she looks, and all she'll hear is a waterfall.

After ten to fifteen minutes, Gail will no longer be able to tell if her eyes are open or closed. Combined with the unpatterned noise she's hearing, this condition will stimulate her brain to provide something more interesting. Many people in the ganzfeld condition describe a pleasant, dreamy, visionary state of awareness.

After being allowed to relax in this dreamlike reverie for a while, Gail is asked to speak aloud anything that comes to mind over the next thirty minutes, while the "sender," Tom, at a distance and strictly isolated from Gail, mentally tries to send a target image to her. In many modern ganzfeld experiments, Gail's utterances are audio recorded so her verbal impressions can be played back to her while she's judging the four target possibilities. This is useful because most people can't clearly remember their impressions after they are taken out of the ganzfeld environment, similar to how memories of dreams quickly fade when you wake up.

The rest of the test we've already described. By pure chance, Gail would be expected to select the correct target first one in four times, for a 25 percent hit rate. If she does better than that, and our experimental controls are in place, then we have evidence that information transferred from Tom to Gail.

Example Session

What follows is a description of a ganzfeld test conducted in our laboratory in September 2010. The participants' real names were Gail and Tom.

Before they came to the lab, a target pool was created consisting of four photos: (1) a grassy field with large yellow and smaller blue flowers; (2) a bird's nest with brown twigs, containing four golden eggs; (3) the great pyramid of Cheops in the Egyptian desert, with two other pyramids in the distance; and (4) a plain asphalt road with a double yellow line going into the distance, with telephone poles on the side of the road, and a flat, barren landscape. The images were kept in separate opaque envelopes, and the target pool was secured so neither Tom nor Gail knew anything about the images.

After they arrived, I explained that after a short guided relaxation period Gail should begin to speak aloud any impressions that came to mind. Her spoken words would be carried by a one-way radio to Tom, who would be located somewhere else at a distance. As part of the protocol, I also told Gail that she should avoid *naming* her impressions. That is, just because she got a flash impression of say, a yellow color, doesn't mean she should automatically assume that the target image was a banana. Past research suggests that this sort of analytical projection is usually wrong, and it tends to override telepathic impressions. So instead, she should try to report perceptual primitives, such as color, shape, and texture.

When the test session began, a research assistant escorted Gail into a heavily shielded room in our laboratory, adjusted the Ping-Pong balls over her eyes, turned on the red light, applied the headphones, and started playing a guided relaxation audio program. While Gail was being set up, I escorted Tom to another room in the building, handed him a die, and asked him to toss it to select one of the four photos in the target pool. He did so. Then after waiting for Gail's relaxation period to finish, I asked Tom to spend the next twenty minutes mentally sending the target image he had selected. He was able to hear Gail's voice over the one-way radio.

What follows is the full transcript of everything that Gail said during that twenty-minute sending period. Each new line indicates a pause. Keep in mind that Gail had no idea what the target was. See if you can guess from her impressions what image Tom had randomly selected.

Keep feeling like looking up at tall, I'm looking up at something tall.
Something about texture. Texture.
I feel like something has a rough texture.
Tall, very tall impression, looking up high.
Feel as if I'm walking around observing something, like when you would walk in an art gallery or in a museum and you would look at something. Wow.
First I'm feeling like tall trees, and then I'm feeling like a tall building and then I'm like a Yosemite kind of image of a tall rock or a tall, some kind of a very tall solid stone something
seeing browns and grays
something like a feeling of walking around, looking up and being in awe, in awe of something.
Monolithic or I don't know what the word is.
I'm getting images of Mount Rushmore, I know you're not supposed to say things.
Half-dome, like just a big stone.
I sort of feel like I'm walking around in a picture, and I'm giving my hand and we're climbing up,
or something about going up, there's . . .
It seems like there's also some kind of a round tall cylinder, and . . .
something long and gray on the right.
Water fountain.
Stone.
At first I felt very much like I was in a nature, forest type of setting, . . .
and now I'm feeling more

something about a, like
a plaza.

When Gail uttered, "I'm getting images of Mount Rushmore, I know you're not supposed to say things," she was referring to my recommendation that she avoid *naming* her impressions.

After the sending period, Gail was shown the four target images and asked to select the one that best matched her experiences. Based on her sense of something tall, an object one might see in a museum, the concept of a monument or monolith, carved rocks, stone, and a plaza, she quickly and confidently selected the photo of the pyramids. In fact, the target that Tom had randomly selected was indeed the photo of the pyramids, so this one test session was a "hit."

This session confirmed to Gail and Tom that their sense of a mental connection between them was real, but of course to anyone else it could easily be regarded as a lucky coincidence. But what if this same test were conducted with hundreds of participants, and it was successfully repeated by dozens of independent laboratories around the world? And what if resolute skeptics who espoused disbelief in telepathy also tried this experiment and obtained similar, positive results? What then?

Multiple Sessions

Psychologists Charles Honorton, William Braud, and Adrian Parker independently developed the ganzfeld technique in the 1970s. These experiments have generated more sustained debate among scientists than any other class of modern psi experiment. An important consequence of all this attention is that this experiment is as close to perfect as anyone has been able to develop. It removes all known biases and clues that might assist the receiver in guessing the target.

Some might argue that this design isn't adequate because it doesn't include a control condition without senders. In such a test Gail would be prepared for the test as usual, but Tom would be asked to engage in some other task completely unrelated to the ganzfeld experiment, and the computer would randomly select the target but not show it to anyone. In that case, Gail should always select the target purely by chance. Right?

Well, no. One problem with a "no sender" design is that it's virtually identical to an experiment in clairvoyance. Also, if Gail's future experience includes an assessment of whether her selection of the target was a hit or miss, it could also be viewed as a test for precognition. But beyond those problems, the ganzfeld test doesn't need a control group. The checks and balances that have evolved to avoid possible design artifacts in these studies are obsessively comprehensive, preventing Gail from obtaining any clue about the target through any normal means. If Gail has no telepathic ability, then on average the absolute best she can do is to achieve a chance hit rate.

Until fairly recently, these experiments were largely unknown outside the rather small discipline of parapsychology. Then, in 1994, psychologists Daryl Bem from Cornell University and Charles Honorton from the University of Edinburgh published a meta-analysis of ganzfeld experiments in the well-regarded journal *Psychological Bulletin*. That article provided strong evidence for a genuine psi effect. Bem and Honorton's review of earlier ganzfeld studies found evidence for telepathy with overall odds against chance of 48 billion to 1, and their review of a series of newly conducted, fully automated experiments that were specifically designed to overcome all known skeptical complaints about the previous studies was also significantly positive, resulting in odds against chance of 517 to 1.

In earlier books, I reviewed the history of the academic debate about the ganzfeld experiment's evidence for telepathy.[1, 2] I showed that all valid critiques about the results of these experiments had been answered through systematic refinements in the methodologies. Hard-nosed skeptics familiar with these studies now agree: There are no known loopholes or flaws that can explain away the results.

From 1974 through 2004, some 88 ganzfeld experiments had been reported. Those studies involved 1,008 hits in 3,145 trials, for a combined hit rate of 32 percent as compared to the chance-expected 25 percent. This 7 percent positive effect would occur by chance with odds of *29 million trillion to 1*. Arguments that this result was due to successful studies being reported more often than unsuccessful studies, the file-drawer effect, have been thoroughly analyzed and reanalyzed over the years. Critics who have studied this literature have agreed that selective reporting does not explain away the positive results.

If we nevertheless insisted that there *had* to be a selective reporting problem, then a conservative estimate of the number of studies needed to nullify the known results is 2,002. That's a ratio of 23 unpublished, unsuccessful studies hidden away for each known study. This means that each of the investigators who conducted these experiments (as of 2004) would have had to conduct but not report an additional 67 studies. Because the average reported ganzfeld study had 36 trials, those estimated 2,002 "missing" studies would have required 67×36 or 72,072 additional test sessions. To produce that many sessions would require an investigator to run ganzfeld sessions twenty-four hours a day, seven days a week, for thirty-six years straight. Not a single one of those hypothetical sessions would ever be published or even known about by any other researcher, and the combined result of all of those sessions would have to produce a flat chance outcome. I suppose it's possible that someone with a massive amount of resources, patience, and determination might have been challenged to take on that Sisyphean task, but it doesn't seem very likely.

When we update the meta-analysis with studies published through 2010, we find 1,323 hits in 4,196 trials, for a combined hit rate of 31.5 percent. The new data increase the overall odds against chance from a mere 29 million trillion to 1 in 2004 to a stunning *13 billion trillion* to 1. This statistical increase is to be expected if telepathy is real, because more data provide an improved statistical ability to detect the effect.

Skepticism

Some may argue that all these experiments were conducted by "believers," and so the credibility of the results might be suspect. What would happen if hard-nosed "disbelievers" conducted these studies? Could they successfully repeat them too, or are the believers allowing their biases to influence the results? There was no answer to this question until recently, because the vast majority of disbelievers are armchair critics. They're adept at offering reasons why they don't believe in something, but they hardly ever bother to put their own beliefs to the test.

This state of affairs changed in 2005.

Two psychologists who explicitly disavowed belief in what they called "psychic powers," Edward Delgado-Romero from the University of Georgia and George Howard from the University of Notre Dame, attempted to replicate the ganzfeld telepathy experiment using the method described above. They published their results in the journal *Humanistic Psychologist.*[240] They wrote:

> After eight studies, we had an overall hit rate of 32% (which agrees with the positive meta-analyses) and, in fact, our hit rate was also statistically significant. . . . (p. 298)

They apparently weren't expecting this positive outcome, so they added their trials to an earlier meta-analysis of ganzfeld studies, published by psychologists Julie Milton and Richard Wiseman, which claimed to show no evidence for telepathy (that analysis was later shown to be flawed, and the actual results *were* successful[241]), whereupon they found that

> [when] our data are added to the Milton and Wiseman (1999) meta-analysis over ganzfeld studies, the overall percent correct responses goes from 26% to 27% and this value now is very close to significant. So, for the moment, even the evidence

against humans possessing psychic powers is precariously close to demonstrating humans do have psychic powers.[240] (p. 298)

At this point, faced with the problem of possibly having to accept the unacceptable, they proposed an ad hoc "psychic theory":

In the ganzfeld procedure, participants are run in pairs. According to psychic theory, if one member of the pair is psychic (P) but the other is not (n) there will be no transmission of information. Only PP [i.e., psychic sender to psychic receiver] pairs can successfully send and receive messages.[240] (p. 298)

Based on this untested theory, they designed an experiment to capitalize on their newly imagined ability to predict when telepathy should occur. They ran the experiment and ended up with too *few* hits, in fact so few that the results were statistically significant in the *negative* direction. From the results of this one pilot test, they reached an astonishing conclusion:

These are enormously disappointing data for individuals who believe humans possess psychic powers—especially because the sample had undergone a selection procedure to increase the percentage of [psychics] in the sample. Due to this last data set, we do not believe that humans possess telepathic powers. Further, the approximately 32% correct figure obtained in an enormous number of psi studies remains perplexing. Perhaps this 7% phenomenon is comparable to Meehl's . . . "crud factor," which suggests that everything is correlated with everything else to a small degree.[240] (p. 300)

In other words, these professors felt more comfortable explaining away thousands of experimental trials reported by investigators around the world, *including their own experiments*, based on a single pilot test, a questionable theory, and the explanatory power of "crud."

First Time Ever

In January 2008, newspapers around the world hailed what was called the first conclusive test for telepathy, conducted by two Harvard University researchers. According to a feature article in the *Boston Globe* newspaper:

> Brain scan tests fail to support validity of ESP. Research on parapsychology is largely taboo in academia, but two Harvard scientists recently set out to settle, once and for all, the age-old question: Is extrasensory perception, or ESP, real? Their sophisticated experiment answers: No, at least, not as far as they can tell using high-tech brain scanners to detect neural evidence of it.[242]

Wow. Once and for all. A sophisticated brain scanner was used to answer the age-old question about telepathy. The high-tech no answer seems conclusive until you read the actual article, which reported that one of the sixteen tests conducted showed a stupendously significant outcome exactly in alignment with what was predicted if psi was in fact real.[243] The authors of the study took great pains to explain why that result was an artifact, or a mistake, and not a psi effect, so the newspapers didn't bother to mention the one intriguing outcome. But it also raises a perplexing question: Why did the authors use a new type of experiment, based on a design that had never been tested before, where the very effect they were looking for could be explained away as a mistake?

Given that this experiment was conducted at Harvard University, the academic equivalent of Mount Sinai as far as most newspaper reporters are concerned, then surely we can now safely close the book on those annoying beliefs about psychic powers. After all, the Harvard scientists used one of those shiny, expensive, brain-scanning machines (the technique is called functional magnetic resonance imaging, or fMRI) to peer deep inside the brain, and they didn't find anything psychic in there. End of story.

Or is it? Was this really the first study to use a functional MRI to investigate psychic abilities? No. It wasn't even the second such study. Or the third. Or fourth. Or fifth. Or sixth. It was the seventh.

And every single one of the other six experiments, all of which were conducted since the year 2000, showed highly significant evidence in favor of psychic phenomena.[190, 244-248] Somehow the Harvard researchers managed to completely overlook all of those studies, and the newspapers didn't bother to check their facts. Four of the seven studies could have been found in a snap by simply searching the National Institutes of Health's online bibliography. The other studies could have been located just as easily by asking researchers who are familiar with this literature.

How is it possible that highly educated scientists, journal referees, and newspaper reporters all failed to notice that the claim of "first time ever" was brazenly wrong, or that the "ESP doesn't exist" conclusion was directly contradicted by a mass of positive experimental evidence? The answer is simple: This study confirmed their prior beliefs, so no one felt it was necessary to check the facts.

Unfortunately, this example is not unique. Bias is pervasive in all human affairs, including science, and it acts like extremely efficient blinders. In the present context, bias within science constrains this type of research from taking place at all. Most funding agencies and foundations, which rely on the expertise of prominent scientists to judge research proposals, are not willing to risk ridicule by supporting studies of phenomena that obviously—so say their experts—don't exist.

Noise Reduction

As previously mentioned, the ganzfeld technique was specifically developed to test a "noise-reduction" model for improving sensitivity to subtle inner impressions, including telepathic impressions. While the evidence for telepathy within the ganzfeld state is clear, those data alone do not allow us to evaluate the noise-reduction concept. Does this idea, based on yogic lore, actually improve psychic functioning?

Over the years there have been many hints that it does, but recently three psychologists, Lance Storm from the University of Adelaide in Australia, and Patrizio Tressoldi and Lorenzo Di Risio from the University of Padua in Italy, analyzed dozens of psi experiments to compare how psychic abilities varied in three types of free-response studies: the ganzfeld telepathy test; other noise-reduction psi tests involving dreams, relaxation, hypnosis, or other techniques; and in experiments using no special methods to alter consciousness.[166] The analysis was published in 2010 in the journal *Psychological Bulletin*.

Storm and his colleagues found in a clearly defined subset of thirty ganzfeld studies that the overall odds against chance were 8.7 billion to 1. The nonganzfeld, noise-reduction experiments showed odds against chance of 4,800 to 1. And experiments with ordinary states of awareness showed odds against chance of 67 to 1. This drop in performance suggested that the ganzfeld experiments produced significantly better performance than ordinary states of awareness and also improved performance (but not in a statistically significant sense) over the nonganzfeld studies. They also found that people selected on the basis of prior experience, prior performance, or meditative experience performed significantly better in the ganzfeld experiments than unselected participants. And they found that these results did not depend on the laboratory that had conducted the studies. The authors concluded, with modest understatement, that

> the noise reduction condition tends to produce stronger effects
> compared with standard free-response studies. . . . In closing,
> we emphasize how important it is to free up this line of investigation from unwarranted skepticism and hasty judgments,
> so that these communication anomalies might be treated and

investigated in like manner with other psychological functions.[166] (p. 480)

Many Meta-Analyses

The first ganzfeld experiments were conducted in 1974. Since then seven meta-analyses have been performed: Two were published in 1985, one in 1994, one in 1999, two in 2001, and the most recent in 2010.[166, 176, 241, 249–252] Meta-analyses usually examine the entire body of experimental data on a given topic, so the later ganzfeld meta-analyses included data from both newly published and previously published studies. Of the seven meta-analyses, six reported statistically significant evidence with odds against chance ranging from a modest 20 to 1 to over a trillion to 1.

All the analysts agreed that the results could not be explained away as artifacts due to selective reporting or to variations in experimental quality. The one and only meta-analysis claiming that the ganzfeld effect had not been demonstrated was published in 1985 by lifelong skeptic Ray Hyman, who, perhaps like Delgado-Romero and Howard, may have been too uncomfortable with the notion of genuine telepathy to allow the published studies to influence his beliefs.[252]

The fact that the other six analyses all showed statistically significant, positive evidence, including one coauthored by well-known British skeptic Richard Wiseman, is striking. It indicates that telepathy has been successfully repeated in many different laboratories, with different investigators and participants in different cultures, over nearly four decades. Persistent, successful repeatability, including by disbelieving skeptics, is as real as it gets in science.

So something interesting is going on. But how can we begin to understand these effects without doing violence to known physics? The yogic approach to the siddhis offers a clue. Yoga says that the siddhis do not arise as a result of magical fairy dust, but rather because the mind is trained to become progressively more sensitive to the holistic nature of reality that we normally can't apprehend.

That is, telepathy arises not because something is transmitted between Gail and Tom, but because from a holistic perspective the objects we perceive as "Gail" and "Tom" are not as separate as they seem. At a deeper level of reality, there is no separateness, including no isolated Gails and Toms. From that view, Gail can know Tom's mind because a part of Gail is already identical with a part of Tom.

Bayesian Analyses

Besides development of ideas that may one day explain telepathy in scientific terms, another advancement in telepathy research is the use of more persuasive ways of analyzing the data. Psychologist Patrizio Tressoldi examined the ganzfeld studies and several other classes of psi experiments using *Bayesian* techniques, which we encountered in the previous chapter on precognition. Tressoldi published his results in 2011 in the journal *Frontiers in Psychology*.[253] He pointed out that the skeptical mantra "Extraordinary claims require extraordinary evidence" contains two perplexing problems. First, how do we know when the evidence we've produced is sufficiently extraordinary to be persuasive, and second, who would be convinced by extraordinary evidence? These questions ultimately rest upon subjective opinions and beliefs, which is what Bayesian statistics are designed to address.

Tressoldi found that in a collection of 108 ganzfeld studies, involving a total of 3,650 participants, a conservative Bayesian analysis resulted in odds against chance of 12 billion to 1. The "Bayes factor," or ratio between the odds in favor of the telepathy hypothesis versus the no-telepathy hypotheses, was 18.8 million to 1 in favor of telepathy. As a rule of thumb, a Bayes factor greater than 100 to 1 is considered "decisive."[254]

By this criterion, there is absolutely no question that the evidence provided by the ganzfeld telepathy studies *should* decisively and rationally bend one's opinion favorably toward the existence of telepathy. Whether it does or not is another matter, as we shall see.

A second class of studies examined by Tressoldi was the presentiment experiments, discussed in the previous chapter. A conservative analysis of thirty-seven presentiment studies resulted in odds against chance of 1.5 billion to 1 and a Bayes factor of 29 trillion to 1 in favor of presentiment.

A third class was two collections of free-response precognitive remote viewing experiments, also discussed in the previous chapter. Those data sets resulted in odds against chance of 6.7 billion to 1 in the first case[182] and 166 million to 1 in the second,[255] along with a Bayes factor of 25 billion to 1. These three classes of studies leave no doubt that these classes of evidence are extraordinary if they are evaluated rationally.

At this point it may seem as though Bayesian methods are magically able to see positive evidence even where there isn't any. But that's not the case. For example, Tressoldi examined several other classes of experiments with Bayesian techniques, and the results were not positive. Psi experiments conducted with altered states of consciousness *other* than the ganzfeld resulted in a Bayes factor of just 0.05. This is considered negative evidence; that is, the evidence supports the null hypothesis of no psi. Similarly, the Bayes factors for psi experiments conducted in normal states of consciousness also supported the null hypothesis. So there is no magic happening here.

Tressoldi concluded that after analyzing several classes of psi experiments, involving more than six thousand participants in over two hundred studies and using both conventional (known as "frequentist") and Bayesian statistics, the results were indeed extraordinary by any reasonable criterion.[253] If studies resulting in combined odds against chance in the millions to trillions to one are not extraordinary enough, then what standard can possibly suffice?

Telepathy in the Wild

A series of clever experiments designed by British biologist Rupert Sheldrake, and conducted since 2003, involved tests for telepathic connections outside the laboratory. These studies used telephones,[256, 257] SMS text messaging,[258] e-mails,[259] and web browsers,[260, 261] to facilitate ways of testing people for telepathy as they went about their daily lives.

The combined odds against chance for these studies are beyond 10^{34} to 1 (that's a 10 followed by 34 zeros). Most of these experiments were open to the public and did not control against cheating, so some of these statistical results may be inflated. However, some of the tests were followed up by retesting participants under conditions with strict controls in place against cheating, such as by videotaping each test session, and the results of those tests showed similar outcomes.[257]

Summary

Telepathy tests developed over many decades have evolved into experiments that are as close to perfect as anyone has been able to devise so far. The results indicate that the likelihood that telepathy exists is as close to "proven" as contemporary science can establish.

We saw in the last chapter that Patanjali was correct about the siddhi of precognition. The same appears to be the case about telepathy. What about his claims for mind-matter interactions?

CHAPTER 11

Psychokinesis in Living Systems

Perhaps the only limits to the human mind are those we believe in.

—*Willis Harman*

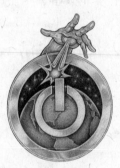

Some of the siddhis in the *Yoga Sutras* are described as interactions between mind and matter, or psychokinesis. *Vibhuti Pada* III.23 suggests that the act of cultivating loving-kindness may have a fieldlike influence whereby one's intentions will affect the mood, attention, or behavior of people in the vicinity. Sutra III.38 is about the power to influence others. III.39 and III.42 are about levitation, and III.44–45 involves mastery over the elements.

In contrast to siddhis having to do with exceptional ways of gaining knowledge through clairvoyance, which are at the top of the list of siddhis, most of the siddhis involving mind-matter interaction are near the bottom of the list. This could be interpreted to mean that they are more advanced abilities, and thus fewer people may be able to master them.

One of the more dramatic claims for the psychokinetic siddhis is levitation. There are numerous historical anecdotes of people who could supposedly do this, sometimes at will, such as yogis and physical mediums, and sometimes spontaneously, like a number of the Catholic saints. Some of them also reportedly had complete mastery of matter. Swami Rama writes in *Living with the Himalayan Masters*:

> I had never before seen a man who could sit still without blinking his eyelids for eight to ten hours, but this adept was very unusual. He levitated two and a half feet during his meditations. We measured this with a string which was later measured by a foot rule. I would like to make it clear, though, as I have already told you, that I don't consider levitation to be a spiritual practice. It is an advanced practice of pranayama with application of *band has* (locks). One who knows about the relationship between mass and weight understands that it is possible to levitate, but only after long practice. . . .
>
> He [also] had the power to transform matter into different forms, like changing a rock into a sugar cube. One after another the next morning he did many such things. He told me to touch the sand—and the grains of sand turned into almonds and cashews. I had heard of this science before and knew its basic principles, but I had hardly believed such stories. I did not explore this field, but I am fully acquainted with the governing laws of the science.[145] (p. 2560)

Levitation

I'm reading a book about anti-gravity. I can't put it down.

In the modern era, the most determined and enthusiastic public attempts to demonstrate levitation were promoted by the Transcendental Meditation (TM) organization. In 1976, it launched the TM-Sidhi program, which promised to train people to perform various siddhis, including "yogic flying." For years TM heavily promoted yogic-flying Olympiads as public relations efforts. In a six-hundred-page coffee-table-style book published in 2008, entitled *The Complete Book of Yogic Flying*, this history is recounted in exquisite detail, accompanied by hundreds of exciting color photos of yogic fliers.[262]

What we see in those photos is not flying. Instead we see people in various stages of hopping, usually with the camera shot frozen at the height of the hop to give the impression that the meditators sitting in lotus positions are hovering in midair. Some historical cases of reported levitation are presented in the book, but what is conspicuously missing is any evidence that levitation was definitively achieved by anyone engaged in the TM-Sidhi practice, or by anyone else in modern times under scientifically controlled conditions.

Yogic flying is described as a process with three stages of development, the first of which is hopping. An explanation for the lack of evidence for the latter two stages—hovering and flying—is offered in a short sidebar near the back of the book. The sidebar title asks, "What will it take for Yogic Flyers to float in the air?" The answer:

In one of his Global Press Conferences, a reporter asked Maharishi, "What will it take for the Yogic Fliers to float in the air, the second stage, and fly through the air, the third stage?" Maharishi replied: "Coherence in the world consciousness. It is the lack of coherence in the world consciousness that doesn't allow the flight to be higher. But as the world consciousness is more and more coherent, flights will be any height, any height. Any height means *any height*. The only limitation comes from the dirty atmosphere around in the collective world consciousness. But it's completely within our reach today. Soon we will have established a reserve fund, the interest from which will be enough to engage sufficient Yogic Flying Vedic Pandits to permanently maintain coherence in world consciousness."[262] (p. 553)

Perhaps this is so, but that reply was provided in 2003 and we are still waiting. In the meantime, the TM program's emphasis on this particular siddhi was, in hindsight, questionable. As Philip Goldberg writes in *American Veda*,

in terms of public perception . . . TM sacrificed much of the respectability it had worked to acquire. Prominent supporters were so embarrassed that they severed their ties. Then came another controversial claim. TM scientists predicted that if the square root of one percent of a population engaged in yogic flying, peace and harmony would reign.[51] (p. 170)

Consciousness Field Effects

The peace and harmony claim in the preceding quote, which was labeled the "Maharishi effect," may be interpreted as a field effect associated with Sutra III.23, the effects of cultivating loving-kindness, or Sutra III.38, the power to influence others, or Sutra II.35, that hostilities cease in the presence of one established in nonviolence.

Unlike with yogic flying, the TM researchers conducted numerous experiments to see if TM-Sidhi practitioners meditating on peace and nonviolence would indeed lower crime, violence, and other acts of aggression in the local area. Perhaps the best known of these studies was an experiment to see if meditators could reduce violent crime in Washington, DC, in June and July 1993.

The study was published in 1999 in the well-regarded journal *Social Indicators Research*.[263] This was a prospective study, meaning it was planned and approved in advance. Two dozen university sociologists and criminologists, representatives from the police department and government of the District of Columbia, and local civic leaders participated in the planning and approval process.

Violent crime was measured by a standard report obtained from the District of Columbia Metropolitan Police Department. As a control comparison, they used data from those same reports for the same two months from the preceding five years (1988–1992). They also tracked variables known to influence violent crime, including changes in weather, changes in police and community anticrime activities, prior crime trends in DC, and crime trends in neighboring cities.

When the researchers analyzed the data after controlling for all known moderating variables, they found a highly significant decrease in violent crimes, and as they had also predicted, the decrease was correlated with an increase in the size of the group of meditators. The maximum decrease was a 23.3 percent reduction in crime as compared to the same period in previous years. The reported odds against chance for this outcome were 500 million to 1.

That sounds impressive, and other TM experiments testing the same idea in different contexts have shown similar outcomes. But critics argued that there were no plausible explanations for how this could have occurred, so it must have been a fluke or due to undiscovered mistakes or statistical problems. These are, of course, exactly the same arguments used to dismiss research on telepathy and precognition, so we are justified in regarding such critiques with skepticism.

Still, TM's emphasis on Vedic philosophy, which is not well known to Western-trained scientists, persuaded many who heard of this study to assume that it was really a religious effort in disguise, and not a valid experiment. As a result, this line of research, which carries huge implications if true, has been essentially ignored by mainstream science.

Intentional Influence at a Distance

If the TM research was the only source of evidence suggesting that collective intentions can influence others at a distance, then that data would be interesting but concerns about their quasi-religious motivations would continue to simmer. Fortunately, there are completely independent experiments, conducted in entirely secular contexts, showing similar effects.

Before discussing those experiments, it is instructive to consider an individual case of the power of "radiated nonviolence." Paul Ekman is a prominent American psychologist who pioneered the analysis of micromovements in facial expressions. In his 2008 book, *Emotional Awareness*,[264] coauthored with the Dalai Lama, Ekman discussed how he was healed from a long-term problem with anger just by being in the presence of the Dalai Lama. Ekman wrote:

I had a very strong physical sensation for which we do not have an English word—it comes closest to "warmth," but there was no heat. It certainly felt very good, and like nothing I have felt before or after. . . . As a scientist, I cannot ignore what I experienced. . . . I think the change that occurred within me started with that physical sensation. I think that what I experienced was—a non-scientific term—"goodness." Every one of the other eight people I interviewed [who reported similar experiences] said they felt goodness; they felt it radiating and felt the same kind of warmth that I did. I have no idea what it is or how it happens, but it is not my imagination. Though we do not have the tools to understand it, that does not mean it does not exist.[264] (p. 229)

Astonished at his response to the presence of the Dalai Lama, Ekman continued to investigate this phenomenon, which he mentioned in a 2009 interview with psychologist David Van Nuys. When asked about his as-yet unpublished study, he replied:

> The only thing that we carried to completion was a study of a single Buddhist monk, who's been a monk for 32 years. And what we were able to do is to identify the differences between different forms of meditation and its impact on his mental state, and we were also able to show the calming effect that his presence had in discussion with people who are normally or typically very aggressive.

Let's turn now to published studies. The first class of experiments examined whether one person's intention can influence a distant person's physiological condition. Another class studied whether one person's intention can modulate a distant person's capacity to concentrate. A third has studied whether there is a global effect associated with large-scale events that capture the simultaneous attention of millions of people.

The first class, known generically as experiments on "distant intentionality," has been repeated some four dozen times by laboratories around the world. In one variation, a person tries to activate or calm the nervous system of a distant, isolated person. In this design, a "sender" gazes at the live video image of a "receiver," providing a formal way of conducting a test of the "feeling of being stared at." In these studies the remote person has no idea when the intention periods occur, or how long they will last. The measurements of interest in most of these studies are physiological indicators of sympathetic nervous system activity, usually measured in the form of skin conductance or heart rate.

In 2004, psychologist Stefan Schmidt and his colleagues from the University of Freiburg Hospital, Germany, published a meta-analysis of all known distant intentionality and distant staring experiments in the *British Journal of Psychology*.[194] In a total of fifty-one studies conducted between 1977 and 2000 by multiple laboratories, involving some 1,394 pairs of participants tested in individual sessions, the combined odds against chance were 15,600 to 1.

Schmidt concluded, with proper scientific caution, that "there is a small, but significant effect. This result corresponds to the recent findings of studies on distant healing and the 'feeling of being stared at.' Therefore, the existence of some anomaly related to distant intentions cannot be ruled out."[194]

The Love Study

Based on Schmidt's findings and our previous studies examining similar effects in the laboratory, our team decided to study the roles of motivation and attention training on this effect.[265] We focused on distant healing because it provided a straightforward way to involve the factor of motivation.

We dubbed the experiment the "Love Study," partially because it was funded by the Institute for Research on Unlimited Love (at the time located at the School of Medicine of Case Western Reserve University), and because an important element of the study focused on cultivating and sending compassionate intention to another person at a distance. This practice is refined to a high art in Tonglen meditation, from the Tibetan Buddhist tradition.

The other important factor in the study was motivation, and healing is a particularly strong motivator. A 2004 government survey of adult Americans, conducted by the United States National Center for Health Statistics, showed that of the top ten complementary and alternative medicine healing practices, the most popular was prayer for self and the second most popular was prayer for others.[266]

Among social workers, a survey found that 28 percent of over two thousand respondents had engaged in verbal prayer with their clients, while 57 percent privately prayed for their clients.[267] In a survey among nineteen hundred cancer survivors, 62 percent reportedly prayed for their own health, 39 percent had others pray for their health, and 15 percent participated in group prayer.[268] And based on general population surveys from 2002 to 2008, the use of prayer for health concerns has continually increased in the United States after taking into account demographics, socioeconomic status, health status, and lifestyle behaviors.[269]

From a psychological perspective, praying for oneself may be thought of as a reasonable coping mechanism in the face of uncertainty and dire need. That prayer for oneself promotes one's own healing is not considered controversial because of the growing literature on the salutary effects of meditation and placebo. Prayer for others is likewise understandable as a practical coping mechanism. But the idea that prayer might actually affect a distant person in any way remains highly contentious.

To avoid unnecessary religious implications in our study, we used the neutral phrase "distant healing intention." Such effects are considered scientifically implausible by some because the term "distant" in distant healing intention means shielded from all known causal interactions.[270] Science is slowly beginning to understand the concept of "spooky action at a distance" within quantum physics, and it is cautiously toying with the idea that *nonlocal* effects might also exist in living systems.[271] But the idea that nonlocal connections might be pragmatically *useful* evokes as much contempt among the orthodox as it does serious interest.

As a short aside, it is useful to know that there are a variety of technical definitions for the term "nonlocal" within physics, but the basic concept is straightforward. Everyday common sense tells us that physical objects interact by bashing into each other. By contrast, *fields*, like gravity, do not seem to follow this simplistic idea, but fields too eventually came to be interpreted as forces carried by particles traveling at the speed of light. Within classical physics the idea of fields and forces seemed to describe just about everything. Everything, that is, except some peculiarities about the nature of light. To gain a deeper understanding of light, quantum mechanics was developed, and out of that our understanding of basic physical concepts like force and causality went through a radical transformation. To trace this history in detail would require a major diversion from the discussion at hand, so let's just say that a nonlocal effect is an interaction that does not involve force, nor does it involve the transfer of signals, and it happens instantaneously regardless of the distance between the objects. *Instantaneously* does not mean faster than the speed of light; rather, it means without any time passing at all. Later in this book we will return to quantum concepts, which can be difficult to grasp because they strongly violate common sense.

Because the mechanisms underlying the postulated effects are unknown, most of these experiments have focused on a straightforward empirical question: *Does it work?* Can distant healing intention really affect medical symptoms and outcomes? Some clinical studies of hospital inpatients and medical outpatients suggest that it might be medically useful,[272] but as a whole the clinical evidence remains uncertain.

For example, in one meta-analysis of seventeen randomized controlled studies of distant healing intention, the conclusion was that the outcomes produced small but significant effects for intercessory prayer.[273, 274] Another meta-analysis that examined fifteen studies that specifically involved intercessory prayer found a positive but statistically nonsignificant outcome.[275] That study also showed that the effect size, while small, was nearly fifteen times larger for unhealthy patients than for healthy controls, suggesting that motivation to be healed may play a role in distant healing efficacy. Nevertheless, because the overall results of these meta-analyses were not robust, the analysts concluded their reports by recommending that further resources not be allocated for this type of research.

The most recent meta-analysis, a systematic review published in 2011,[276] found fewer deaths in a prayer condition as compared to standard care control, results that were very significant for high-risk, highly motivated patients (odds against chance were greater than 100,000 to 1). But the conclusion of that analysis was curiously pessimistic: "The evidence presented so far is interesting enough to support further study. However, if resources were available for such a trial, we would probably use them elsewhere" (p. 24).[276]

For pragmatic reasons that conclusion is not unreasonable. Funds available for research are always limited, so effects that cannot be easily explained rarely attract financial support. In any case, the conclusion for distant healing intention tested under controlled laboratory conditions is more optimistic than the clinical trials. The laboratory evidence may be clearer because there are no "competing" intentions to interfere with the test results, such as the prayers of clinical patients' loved ones who are not part of the formal test. It is also clearer because physiological fluctuations can be objectively monitored in real time, whereas healing responses in the clinic may progress over days or weeks.

However, the context of laboratory studies is also dramatically different from that of clinical studies. In the lab, the person assigned to "send" the distant healing intention (hereafter called the *sender*) is typically a volunteer who is not especially motivated or trained, and the person assigned to receive distant healing intention (the *receiver*) is often just curious to see what will happen.

The goal of our Love Study was to see what would happen when powerful, real-life motivations associated with clinical trials were combined with the controlled context and objective measures offered by laboratory protocols. We were also interested in seeing whether motivation and meditative training would enhance the effect by recruiting long-term, emotionally bonded couples, friends, and family members. Given the laboratory context, we were not testing distant *healing* per se, but rather the physiological effects of one person's intention on a distant person.

Design

Two of the groups that we recruited were adult couples, one of whom was healthy and the other was undergoing treatment for cancer. The healthy partner was assigned the role of the *sender* and the patient the role of the *receiver*. In a "trained group," we invited the sender to attend a program involving discussion and the practice of cultivating compassionate intention, which was defined as the act of directing selfless love toward another person with the intention to relieve their suffering and enhance their well-being.

The meditation training program was a daylong, eight-hour group workshop. The sender was instructed to practice the meditation daily for a half hour for three months, and then those couples were tested in the laboratory. In a "wait group," the couple was tested before the healthy partner attended the training program. A third, control group, consisted of healthy couples who received no training.

When a couple arrived at the lab, we attached electrodes to each person to monitor skin conductance and other variables including heart rate and respiration. The couple was asked to maintain a "feeling of connectedness" with each other at all times during the experiment. To assist with this intentional focus, each person was asked to exchange a personal item, like a ring or watch, and to hold that object in a free hand for the duration of the test session. In the control group, couples were asked to decide which of the two might be more receptive, and that person was assigned the role of the receiver. In the trained and wait groups, the receiver was always the cancer patient.

Environment

The receiver was asked to relax in a reclining chair inside our lab's double-steel-walled, electromagnetically shielded chamber. The receiver was informed that the sender would be viewing his or her live video image at random times from a distant location, and that during those periods the sender would make a special intentional effort to mentally connect with him or her. At other times the video image would be switched off and the sender would just relax and stop sending intention.

No one involved in the experiment knew exactly when these periods would occur, as they were timed by a computer, and the receivers also did not know how long these intentional or relaxation periods would last. The actual times were ten seconds for the intentional periods, with a randomly determined epoch of five to forty seconds between those periods.

As in any experiment investigating connections at a distance, we had to be sure that no ordinary forms of information could pass between the couple, so we tested for possible sensory cues by blasting tones as loud as 110dB in the sender's room to see if it could be detected inside the receiver's shielded chamber. We used a Coast Guard air horn for these tests, and the sound was so loud that we accidentally summoned the local fire department, located several miles away, because they thought they heard a fire alarm.

We conducted both subjective hearing tests and tests using a digital sound-level meter, and we confirmed that the Coast Guard sound blasts were indistinguishable from background noise inside the chamber. So ordinary sounds could not leak into the chamber to provide clues for the receiver. To further isolate the shielded room from potential infrasound or vibration cues, the testing chamber rested on a vibration-dampening mat on a concrete floor.

After the receiver was settled comfortably in the shielded room, the sender was led through two closed doors to a dimly lit room twenty meters away and asked to sit in a chair in front of a video monitor.

Results

Thirty-six couples participated in the study. Analysis of the senders' skin conductance levels across all participants showed that it increased substantially *after* the receivers' images appeared on the video screen.

This was expected because it confirmed that the senders' sympathetic nervous system became activated as a result of their increased mental effort associated with sending distant healing intention. As shown in Figure 7, about two seconds after the video switched on, the senders' average skin conductance (this is also called electrodermal activity, or EDA) began to increase, peaking about three seconds later.

In statistical terms, the rise in the sender's skin conductance was associated with odds against chance of more than 10^{32} to 1 (that's a 10 with 32 zeros after it), so it is absolutely certain that as a group the senders were actively engaged in doing something, hopefully the assigned task. This large difference also established that as a group the senders had not fallen asleep during the experiment (which can happen).

The more interesting question is what was happening to the receivers, who were resting comfortably in the shielded chamber. The data showed that their skin conductance also significantly increased shortly after the senders saw their video image (the bold line in Figure 7), reaching its peak value by the time the video switched off ten seconds later. The peak was associated with odds against chance of 21,000 to 1.

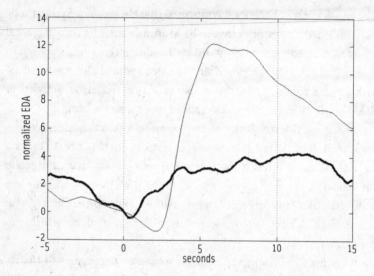

Figure 7. Sender (thin line) and Receiver (bold line) normalized mean electrodermal activity (EDA) across all 38 test sessions (N = 1,104 epochs), from 5 seconds before stimulus onset (at 0 seconds on the x-axis) to 5 seconds after stimulus offset (at 10 seconds) to show the effect in context.

Comparison of the receiver's skin conductance across the three groups revealed an interesting trend, as shown in Figure 8. Receivers in all three groups responded quickly at the start of the sending period, but the control group's reactions subsided after four seconds, the wait group's reaction was initially stronger but subsided after five seconds, and the trained group's reaction continued to rise progressively for eight seconds, finally reaching the maximum deviation among all three groups. This suggests that both the sender's meditation training and motivation enhanced the receiver's response over motivation alone, and motivation enhanced the response over interest alone.

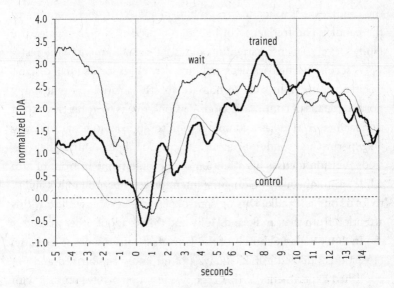

Figure 8. Comparison of receivers' skin conductance levels in the three groups.

Distant Facilitation

So far, we've discussed evidence indicating that one person's intention can influence the physiology of a distant person, and that the intentions of trained meditators have a somewhat larger effect than non-meditators. Through the TM-Sidhi program we found that meditators' intentions may affect the behavior of the local population as measured through reduced indices of violence. A third class of studies, called the "attention focusing facilitation" design, takes a variation of the TM-Sidhi claim into a controlled laboratory context to see if one person's focused attention can remotely help a distant person to focus his or her attention.

In a "distant facilitation of attention" experiment, the distant person—let's call her Holly—is asked to focus her attention on a candle flame. As soon as Holly notices that her mind is wandering from the candle, she is asked to press a button and return her attention to the candle. The frequency of her button presses is used to measure Holly's level of focused attention and is the measurement of interest.

A second participant, let's call him Vernon, is located in a distant, isolated room. Holly and Vernon are strictly isolated to exclude any normal means of communication. Vernon's role is to act as the "attention facilitator." He has a computer monitor in front of him displaying an experimental condition, either "control" or "help." During help periods, Vernon focuses his attention on a candle flame in front of him while simultaneously holding the intention to enhance Holly's ability to focus on her candle. During control periods, Vernon withdraws his attention from the candle and Holly and thinks about other matters.

In 2010, Stefan Schmidt of the University of Freiburg (Germany) Hospital conducted a meta-analysis of all known published and unpublished experiments of this type.[277] He found twelve studies with nearly identical designs conducted between 1993 and 2006. One study was excluded because of possible artifacts identified by the original investigators. For the remaining eleven experiments, consisting of 576 individual test sessions, Schmidt calculated an effect size of 0.11, which was associated with odds against chance of 100 to 1. This provides modest evidence that remote facilitation of attention may be possible, and the results are consistent with the other forms of distant influence that have been studied.

Summary

The psychokinesis studies discussed in this chapter provide evidence for mind-matter interactions, but the cause of those interactions can be interpreted in two principal ways. One way to generate a physiological response in a receiver's body is through application of force, like poking the receiver with a stick. The second way is by gently whispering, "You've just won the lottery." The first case is suggestive of a mind-body interaction involving a distant *force* or influence from the sender. The second case is suggestive of a mind-to-mind interaction, an *informational* exchange that hardly involves any force. With this class of studies it isn't possible to tell with certainty which explanation is better. Thus, to explore mind-matter interactions where mind-to-mind influences are excluded, let's consider experiments involving nonliving targets of intention.

CHAPTER 12

Psychokinesis in Inanimate Systems

To see a thing clearly in the mind makes it begin to take form.
—*Henry Ford, in* Theosophist Magazine, *February 1930*

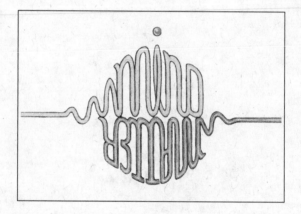

Experiments investigating mind-matter interactions have explored many types of inanimate physical targets, ranging from objects that are big enough to see with the naked eye (known as "macro-PK" targets) to objects or systems that are microscopic (known as "micro-PK" targets).

The target system that has been used in the vast majority of psychokinetic studies is the behavior of random physical systems. This has proven to be a useful micro-PK target because it is assumed that to influence, say, a photon bouncing off versus passing through a half-silvered mirror, or the time between successive decays of radioactive particles, would require an extremely small amount of force; metaphorically speaking, dramatic changes in such systems would only require the touch of a feather. Randomness is also a convenient target because the statistics of random variables are well understood. This makes evaluating the data in these experiments simple and easy. But let's begin our investigation by considering macro-PK targets.

Macro-PK

Mentally bending cutlery or aluminum bars has been informally tested many times in so-called PK parties, a lighthearted party game originally designed by Jack Houck, an aeronautical engineer. These parties were originally stimulated by displays of apparent psychokinetic "spoon bending" in the 1970s by the Israeli psychic Uri Geller. This phenomenon has been studied a few times under quasi-controlled circumstances, and in my opinion, it seems like something interesting may be going on. However, because there are many clever ways of bending metal using conjuring techniques, from a scientific perspective the evidence is insufficient and so the jury is out.

That said, if I were forced to decide whether it was *possible* to bend metal for real, without using blunt force or conjuring methods, then I would say yes, it is possible. I've seen it performed up close both by magicians who were faking it, and by ordinary people who were not faking it. If I only had those two categories of evidence on which to base my decision, I would be less certain. But I've also done it myself, and I know that what I did wasn't a trick.

Here's what happened: I was attending a PK party with the

intention of carefully watching a woman who claimed to have previously bent the bowl of a soup spoon. I too was holding a large, heavy soup spoon, mimicking her hand movements to get a better feel for what she might have been doing.

While watching her intensely, I heard someone shout, "Look what you've done!" I looked up to see what the commotion was about, and someone said no, look at what *I* had done. I had somehow bent the bowl of the spoon I was holding about 90 degrees. I immediately checked my fingers to see if I had unconsciously used force, because it would have taken an enormous effort to create that bend and the effort would have left clear indentations on my fingers. There were no signs of force.

Then someone shouted, "Bend it all the way!"

To my surprise the bowl felt soft, like putty, so I pinched it with a thumb and forefinger. After the bowl folded over, it stiffened, and within a few seconds it became as hard as steel. The spoon felt cool to the touch, the bent portion was shiny smooth, and there were no signs of metal fatigue. I still have that spoon sitting on my shelf; it mocks me every time I glance at it, and it reminds me about a peculiar experience that I might have otherwise suppressed.

Later I tested if I could achieve the same bend on the same model spoon without causing damage to my fingers or hands. I couldn't budge it, regardless of how hard I tried. I suppose it's possible that metal can behave strangely under certain conditions that might be catalyzed by handling, but I've never seen a piece of cutlery act that way in ordinary use, from freezing cold to boiling hot, or with shallow or heavy pressure. Nor have I been able to repeat the effect. So I can't explain *how* this happened, nor do I present it as evidence for macro-PK. But it did happen.

Moving Objects

A second category that has not been tested in any systematic, scientifically rigorous way are psychokinetic targets in the form of thin metal foil or paper pinwheels balanced on a pin, or paper spirals hanging from a thread, or movement of small objects like a Ping-Pong ball floating in water or a bit of crumbled-up paper. All these are very popular targets among amateur enthusiasts, and there are hundreds of videos on YouTube where people display their supposed skills. I have yet to find any of these cases that have been properly studied under conditions that strictly exclude mundane influences.

That said, I do know of a few cases where the claimant is sincere, and where small but visible movements do occur under fairly well-controlled conditions. So the possibility remains that there *might* be genuine mind-matter interactions going on. To know for sure, the test setup would have to exclude artifacts that can mimic PK effects, including convection currents in the air caused by the heat of the hands, force fields from static electricity, vibrations due to proximity of and movements by the body, air flow caused by breathing, and so on. Establishing such controls is possible, but to do it right wouldn't be cheap.

Teleporting Objects

Another source of remarkable claims about macro-PK comes from China. In China, psi research translates roughly into "Exceptional Functions of the Human Body," and reports of highly accurate psi effects, including clairvoyance and psychokinetic effects, have been common since the 1970s.

In a report published in 2010 by Dong Shen, a retired research chemist, an experiment is described involving mental teleportation of bits of paper out of a sealed plastic film container.[278] This is quite a claim, but even more amazing is that this skill was reportedly trained. The technique is called the development of the "second consciousness state," and the contention of the researchers who have been study-ing this technique is that this method has been taught to hundreds of people with a 40 percent success rate.[279] Unfortunately, evaluating the details and credibility of these studies has been difficult because many of the papers appear only in Chinese, the techniques have not yet been repeated outside of China, and the experimental methods employed in conducting such tests do not appear to be as rigorously controlled as compared to typical Western methods.

. . .

The bottom line about macro-PK is that the jury is out. We don't have enough data collected under sufficiently strict controls to gain much confidence about mind-matter interactions large enough to be seen with the naked eye. The yogic lore tells us that it is possible, but so far science, at least as practiced in the West, is uncertain.

This, however, is not the case for small-scale psychokinetic effects.

Micro-PK

Consider an experiment entitled "Quantum-Mechanical Processes and Consciousness," conducted by neuroscientist Lawrence Farwell and physicist George Farwell and presented at a 1995 meeting of the American Physical Society.[280, 281] Their study was described as follows:

> We investigated the possible effect of human consciousness and intention on a quantum-mechanical process. The experi-mental apparatus consisted of a small natural alpha-particle source, a solid-state particle detector, amplifiers, a single-channel analyzer and pulse shaper, an oscilloscope, and a com-puter with digitizer board. Count rates of about 1 kHz were observed, and the intervals (in [microseconds]) between suc-

cessive alpha-decay events were sensed and recorded. Without outside influence, one predicts 50% even and 50% odd time intervals for successive particle detections.

Acting over a succession of 10-[second] intervals randomly assigned to the 3 below conditions, the 23 experimenters, all experienced in achieving advanced states of consciousness, attempted to influence the decay process so as to yield (1) an excess of intervals of an even number of [microseconds] ("even events"); (2) an excess of "odd events"; or (3) either (control condition). In 11,721,660 events in the "even" and "odd" conditions, we observed a total excess of 12,176 in the intended direction (i.e., "even" where intended and "odd" where intended), [associated with odds against chance of 5,000 to 1]. (In the control condition the numbers of "even" and "odd" events were statistically indistinguishable.)[281] (pp. 956–57)

While Lawrence Farwell was justifiably pleased with this outcome, his later description of this study was overly enthusiastic. He wrote, "I have now collected the data necessary to reach a definite conclusion: consciousness can and does command matter at the quantum-mechanical level" (p. 5).[280] This was too confident because, as I've previously mentioned, a single experiment cannot provide a *definitive* result. For that kind of confidence we need to see successful repetitions by many different laboratories.

For micro-PK effects we have that kind of evidence. In spades.

Random Number Generators

Farwell's experiment was a replication of decades of previously reported experiments. The first study testing whether intention could speed up or slow down radioactive decay rates was published by psychologist John Beloff and his colleague Leonard Evans in 1961, when they were at Queen's University, Belfast, Ireland.[282] They measured the decay rates of radioactive alpha particles from uranyl nitrate, and thirty men and women volunteers participated. That study found no evidence for a micro-PK effect.

But shortly after Beloff's study, when electronic circuits and then microprocessors became more readily available, an improved micro-PK experiment was developed by physicist Helmut Schmidt. He created an electronic random number generator (RNG), where the randomness was based on quantum events regarded as fundamentally random; that is, completely unpredictable.

Schmidt's device was essentially an extremely fast coin-flipping system that provided automated recording of the results, and where the coins were, in effect, the behavior of elementary particles, like electrons. As circuitry improved, these RNGs became devices that could be completely controlled by a computer. This allowed for all sorts of clever presentation and feedback techniques. In its modern form, an RNG is a small box powered by and operated through any computer's universal serial bus (USB) connection.

Over the past half century, hundreds of psychokinesis tests using RNGs have been published, and several meta-analyses have summarized the combined results. The most recent meta-analysis was published in 2006 in the journal *Psychological Bulletin* by Holger Bösch from University Hospital in Freiburg, Germany, and his colleagues.[196] (For ease of readability I will refer to this paper as though it was written by Bösch alone.)

In his analysis, Bösch excluded any RNG studies involving (a) indirect or implicit forms of intention, (b) animals, (c) plants, or (d) babies as participants, or the use of (e) hidden RNGs as targets, (f) retrocausal designs studying possible intentional influences from the future, or (g) designs using pseudorandom or algorithmic-based random generators. Studies were also excluded if their (h) outcomes could not be transformed into the effect size that Bösch was using for his analysis. The various exclusions eventually removed over 200 experiments from the published literature, and it resulted in a subset of 380 experiments, all testing whether RNG outputs correlated with human intention.

Bösch's conclusion was that there was "a significant but very small overall effect size," and that selective reporting bias was "the easiest and most encompassing explanation for the primary findings of the meta-analysis."[196]

My colleagues and I had conducted several previous meta-analyses of this same literature, and in our assessment the evidence in favor of a genuine mind-matter interaction effect was much clearer than Bösch's ambivalent conclusion. So I went through his arguments in detail, and I found that we both agreed that the published studies indicated the existence of a genuine psychokinetic effect, that the studies were generally of high methodological quality, and that the effects were distributed heterogeneously, meaning there was a wide range of reported effect sizes. In fact, the only thing that we disagreed on was the source of the heterogeneity.

Bösch proposed that a selective reporting problem was inflating the results of the meta-analysis, and that if those missing studies could be found (he estimated there were 1,544 missing studies), then the overall results would show no evidence for psychokinesis.

Having conducted some of these RNG experiments myself, and knowing most of the other investigators who had contributed similar studies to the literature, I thought it was most implausible that there were as many as 1,544 missing experiments. So I investigated further and discovered why Bösch reached his conclusion: He assumed that the effect size in these studies was independent of the sample size.

This sounds like a complicated statistical issue, but it's really quite simple. Bösch's assumption was incorrect. Here's how my colleagues and I explained it in our response, which was also published in *Psychological Bulletin*.[197]

[Imagine] that we conduct a study involving 1,000 experienced meditators, each of whom is selected on the basis of his or her performance on a previous, similar [psychokinesis] task.

Each participant is asked by a cordial, enthusiastic investigator to engage in a daily intention-focusing practice for 4 weeks in preparation for the experiment, in which he or she will be asked to intentionally influence the generation of a single random bit. Participants are told that the outcome of that random decision will determine the outcome of a meaningful bonus, such as winning a scholarship. Now consider a second study in which a bored student investigator indifferently recruits an arbitrarily selected college sophomore, who is asked to mentally influence 1,000 random bits generated in a millisecond, with no feedback of the results and no consequences regardless of the outcome.

The physical context of these two studies may be identical, using the same [random number generator] and statistics to evaluate the resulting data sets, each of which consists of a total of 1,000 randomly generated bits. But it is clear that the psychological contexts differ radically. If we presume that the only important factor in this type of experiment is the number of bits generated, then the two studies should provide about the same results. But if a significant variable is the amount of time or effort one can apply in focusing mental intention toward each random event, then the former study might result in an effect size orders of magnitude larger than the latter. (p. 529)

Besides the problem with Bösch's initial assumption, we found that he also excluded three very large experiments as "outliers," but those studies had reported highly significant outcomes. Those three studies also contained over 210 times as much data as all the remaining 377 studies combined. In addition, Bösch's assumption that selective reporting could explain away the results was based on a mathematical model with parameters that could be used to fit any desired outcome, so it wasn't a fair approach to estimating the size of the file-drawer effect.

To check Bösch's estimate, we conducted a survey among the researchers who had conducted most of these RNG studies to estimate the actual number of unreported experiments. The answer was "1"; that is, one unreported experiment per investigator. And it wasn't the case that the missing studies were uniformly unsuccessful. Some of them showed significantly positive results.

This suggested that perhaps 59 studies (the same as the number of investigators) were potentially missing from Bösch's database, and not 1,544. If those 59 studies had been found, and every single one of them had ended up with a null outcome (which we knew was not the case), it wouldn't budge the overall results. So Bösch's conclusion that publication bias was the easiest explanation for the meta-analysis was unjustified.

Another critique of the RNG experiments, by Martin Schub,[283] started with the same assumption as Bösch's: The effects in these experiments should be exactly the same for each generated random sample, independent of the number of samples used in an experiment or the rate at which the samples were generated or the psychological conditions of the task. As we said in our response,

> the problem with this assumption is that there is no valid reason to expect that [mind-matter interaction] should behave in this way. Indeed, we are unaware of any sort of human performance that is unaffected by such parametric changes. For example, a factory worker who can identify defective parts with 100% accuracy as they roll by at one or two per second will do no better than chance if the conveyor belt is suddenly accelerated to 1,000 parts per second. And yet the bit rate in the various [random number generator] experiments range over not just three orders of magnitude, but six orders, and they involve significant physical differences in the underlying mechanisms for generating random bits.[284] (p. 362)

Experimenter's Regress

Most scientists would probably agree that demonstrating the existence of a genuine mind-matter interaction effect, regardless of the magnitude of the effect, would be of profound importance. And thus careful consideration of this topic is amply warranted. But different personal beliefs and predilections invariably lead to different assessments of the same evidence. Scientists who worry about accidentally accepting something as true that is actually false (called a Type I error) insist on absolute proof-positive before taking the evidence seriously. Others who are more concerned about accidentally rejecting something as false that is actually true (called a Type II error) prefer to take a more affirmative stance.

The Type I personality is reflected in Bösch's comment that "this unique experimental approach will gain scientific recognition only when we know *with certainty* what an unbiased funnel plot . . . looks like" (p. 517).[196] We find a similar statement in Schub's comment that "*perfect methodological quality* is a logical necessity in parapsychology, since a paranormal effect can only be demonstrated if all possible non-paranormal causes are ruled out" (p. 410).[283]

Demands for perfect, absolutely certain results are unrealistic. Perfection is not practically achievable in any experiment, and when the plea for perfection is unpacked, it's found to contain an irresolvable paradox known as the *experimenters' regress*.[285] This is a catch-22 that arises when the correct outcome of an experiment is unknown. That is, if we want to settle the "Does it exist?" question when the outcome of an experiment is clearly predicted by a well-accepted theory, then the results are simply compared to the prediction. If they match, then we know that the study was conducted properly. If the outcome does not match, then the experiment must have been flawed. This match-mismatch approach is the basis of how most student laboratories are designed. If you obtain the expected results, you are rewarded; if you don't, the results are discarded as mistakes or outliers, and you start over.

Unfortunately, when it comes to pretheoretical concepts, which is always the case at the leading edge of knowledge, to judge whether an experiment was performed "perfectly," or even to know with any degree of certainty what the results are *supposed* to look like, we first need to know whether the phenomenon of interest exists and how it behaves. But to know that, we need to conduct the correct experiment. But to conduct the correct experiment, we need a well-accepted theory to inform us what "correct" means.

You see the problem.

For scientists with Type I temperament, this paradox continues to loop forever. It doesn't matter how rigorous the scientific investigation is—it can never be good enough. The stalemate is broken only by Type II scientists who are willing to entertain the possibility that nature consists of many wonderful phenomena, most of which are not yet understood.

Given the powerful biasing effects of one's adopted beliefs, it is not surprising that scientists mainly tend to perceive their predilections. (There is another, more radical possibility that we will discuss in the last chapter.) Of course, the goal in science is to get beyond personal beliefs and discover the objective truth as best as possible. Skeptical attacks can be irritating, but they are also helpful because they reveal biases on both sides of the debate, and eventually they allow the state of the art to evolve.

Field Consciousness

Because laboratory tests suggest that mind-matter interactions can be detected through the statistical behavior of random events when RNGs are subjected to intention, these same devices can also be used to test the siddhi suggesting fieldlike influences, as described in *Vibhuti Pada* III.23. Such studies, dubbed experiments in "field consciousness," were pioneered in the mid-1990s by Princeton University psychologist Roger Nelson.

The idea of a consciousness field refers to that subjective sense when individual thoughts and actions seem to merge into a single group thought or action. A qualitative sense of this type of coherence is captured in phrases like being "in the zone," or "in the flow," or "on the same wavelength." It is sometimes reported during meaningful religious rituals, at sacred sites, in the midst of emotionally stirring speeches, and when engaged in team sports or singing in choruses. At such times the scattered attentions of individuals seem to lock onto the same wavelength, and people report a sense that something has gelled or shifted inside.

Experiments in field consciousness explore whether such felt shifts are associated with actual physical changes in the local environment. They ask the question, When the "mind" side of a mind-matter interaction relationship becomes unusually coherent, does the "matter" side of that relationship also become more coherent?

To detect the proposed coherence effect, RNGs have been used because they are physical systems designed to produce maximum entropy (randomness), and as such if unexpected moments of order appear, they can be detected in a straightforward statistical manner. The RNG used in a field consciousness experiment generates a continuously recorded sequence of random bits (0s and 1s) while groups are involved in highly engaging activities. In some studies, deviations of these data from chance are compared to chance-based theoretical expectations; in others, a baseline measure of randomness is collected during control periods when no group activity is taking place, and later data collecting during the two conditions are compared. The field consciousness hypothesis in both cases predicts that significantly more statistical order will appear in the experimental data during times of high collective mental coherence.

Let's say that one *sample* in one of these experiments consists of two hundred successive random bits. The chance-expected number of 1s and 0s in each sample, assuming a properly constructed RNG, would be one hundred 1s and one hundred 0s. The type of statistical order we are looking for in these studies would be either more 0s or more 1s than would be expected by chance. The statistic used to measure that type of order is a change in what's called the sample *variance*. If we were only interested in looking at an increase in, say, 1s, then we would look for a change in the sample mean or *average* value. Variance refers to the range or distribution that collections of samples show, rather than the average value of those samples.

Over a hundred field consciousness experiments have been reported.[286–289] The cumulative evidence strongly supports the existence of a genuine effect, with odds against chance far beyond a million to one. But the reported results vary quite a bit. Some portion of that variation is probably due to differences among the group compositions, their activities, the environmental context, and so on, but it may also be due to uncertainty involved in inferring exactly when, or if, mental coherence arises.

The Hemi-Sync Experiment

To explore this issue, I collaborated with Skip Atwater, former president of the Monroe Institute (TMI), to see if TMI's mental coherence-enhancing binaural-beat audio tones known as Hemi-Sync would allow us to more reliably detect a field consciousness effect. "Binaural-beat" refers to a method in which one tone at, say, 400 Hz, is played in one ear while another tone at, say, 406 Hz, is played in the other ear. These two pure tones are heard along with a subjective beat frequency, or warbling tone, generated by overlapping neural circuits in the audio processing regions of the brain's two hemispheres.

The beat frequency entrains the brain's oscillatory rhythm, so in this example the binaural-beat would tend to promote a theta rhythm at 6 Hz.[290, 291] Hemi-Sync audio programs combine the binaural-beat technique along with relaxation techniques, reduced environmental stimulation, controlled breathing, guided affirmations, and visualization. Binaural-beat programs are said to reduce stress and encourage other beneficial physical and mental health outcomes.[292]

In our experiment we focused on a six-day workshop periodically held at the Monroe Institute, known as the Gateway Voyage. In this workshop, groups of twenty to twenty-five people simultaneously listen to a prescribed sequence of Hemi-Sync programs presented over headphones for up to six hours a day, while each person relaxes in his or her own listening chamber.

We speculated that these group listening periods, where each person is being entrained to the same brain rhythms, might produce a form of collective mental coherence, similar to how participating in a drumming ceremony entrains both the drummers and the spectators. In the Gateway Voyage workshop, after the individuals listen to a Hemi-Sync program for about forty-five minutes, the group reassembles and discusses their experiences. This listening-discussing cycle is repeated throughout the day for six days. These workshops always follow the same prescribed sequence of Hemi-Sync audio programs.

Assuming that the field consciousness idea is correct, if group coherence increases while listening to the tones, and it is minimized during breaks and meals and while the workshop participants are sleeping, then similar variations in order ought to appear in the random data from one workshop to the next.

To test this idea, we calculated all the correlations between the RNG-generated data collected in repeated workshops, and we predicted that the average cross-correlation between those data sets would be significantly positive. That is, we predicted that physical randomness would be modulated by the same sequence of mental activities repeated again and again, thereby creating a positive relationship between data sets where by chance one would expect no relationship at all. By contrast, data collected from the same random generators in the same locations, starting at the same time and also running continuously for six days, but without workshops taking place, were predicted not to show any systematic cross-correlations.

All the Gateway Voyage workshops in our study took place in the same location at the Monroe Institute. We also ran RNGs in two distant locations while the workshops were under way. One was in a laboratory about a tenth of a mile away from the workshop location, and the other was about a mile away in a remote building. The distant random generators were in quiet locations away from human activity.

Most of the workshop participants did not know that RNGs were present during these tests, and no one ever obtained any feedback from them while they were operating. Only Skip Atwater knew where they were located. As in all field consciousness experiments, this was not a test of a group's coherent *intentions*, but rather their collective *attention*.

Results

Two of the electronic RNGs that we used for this experiment had been extensively tested and calibrated in previous research; we also used a third, Geiger-counter-based RNG. We collected data from one to three RNGs running continuously and simultaneously during fourteen weekly workshops. Those same RNGs were also run continuously during eight weeks when no workshops were taking place, to provide control data. All together, over the course of this experiment 108 billion random bits were generated and stored.

Analysis showed that the average cross-correlation among all data sets produced by the RNGs during the workshops were significantly positive, as predicted, with associated odds against chance of 500 to 1.[293] The same analysis applied to control data sets showed no effect. Data from the distant RNGs, collected both during the workshops and in the control conditions, also showed no effect. This experiment supported the outcomes of previous studies, suggesting that people engaged in coherence-enhancing activities do modulate physical randomness in the environment.

Global Consciousness Project

The Global Consciousness Project (GCP), directed by Princeton University psychologist Roger Nelson since its inception in 1998, was designed to expand the field consciousness experiment from small groups of people engaged in a common event to periods of global mental coherence generated as a result of major news events that attract worldwide attention.

With the explosion of social networking websites, and a growing number of Internet-based instant news alerts, the GCP proposes that within a few minutes of major events, a sizable fraction of the world's attention orients toward the same topic, and as a result of that global shift and the accompanying mental coherence, RNGs located around the world will all deviate from chance behavior.

The GCP can be thought of as a kind of mental tsunami detection system. Instead of monitoring an ocean of water it monitors an "ocean of consciousness." Imagine a vast ocean with scores of buoys dancing on the waves. Each buoy has a bell attached to it to alert passing ships about hidden reefs and shallows. The sound of each buoy's bell is broadcast by radio to a land-based central receiving station. That station receives all the radio transmissions and consolidates them to form a single collective tone reflecting the ocean's grand dance.

Most of the time this sound is completely unpatterned, similar to the random tinkling one might hear from a set of wind chimes dangling in a breeze. But every so often the buoys mysteriously synchronize and their tones swell into a great harmonic chord. When that occurs, we know that something big has affected the entire ocean.

Buoys reflect movements only on the ocean's surface, and the ocean is complex and deep. So most of the time we can only infer what caused the big event. Possibilities include an earthquake, a meteorite strike, or perhaps something stirring in the ocean's depths. That something might be quite small and subtle at its origin, but if it's deep enough, then by the time it rises to the surface it can become enormously powerful and encompass the entire ocean.

Whatever the cause, we are interested in two types of analyses when the buoys' bells coalesce into a harmonious chord. The first is how loud it is (by analogy, the amplitude of the tone), and the second is how coherent it is (the degree of harmony of the tone).

The GCP's network began with three RNG sites in 1998. Over time, it increased in size as volunteers were found who were willing to host an RNG on their personal computer. After a few years, the network size had stabilized to about sixty-five active RNGs located throughout the world. Each RNG collects one sample (of 200 random bits each) per second, and each sample is time-stamped and synchronized to standard Internet time. Every five minutes, all data in the network is assembled and sent over the Internet to a central web server in Princeton, New Jersey, where it is automatically entered into a massive database.

The data are analyzed in a rigorously predefined way, *before* any of the data are examined, to see whether the streams of random samples generated by the RNGs deviate from chance expectation in certain predefined ways. For most events, the analysis examines data from a few minutes before an event of interest to a few hours afterward. By September 2012, a total of 415 events of global interest had been defined, and the data were analyzed and double-checked by independent analysts. The events included New Year celebrations, natural disasters, terrorist activity, massive meditations, sports events, outbreaks of war, outbreaks of peace, unexpected deaths of celebrities, and so on.

The overall results show an unambiguous deviation from chance, with odds against chance of 284 billion to 1 (see Figures 9–11).[294] This suggests that when a sizable proportion of the planet's population focuses their *mental* attention toward the same event, then the amount of *physical* coherence in the world also increases. These episodes of unusual physical coherence are not just limited to RNG outputs; they would theoretically affect everything, assuming the field consciousness idea is correct.

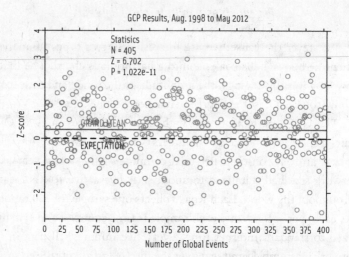

Figure 9. Statistical results of the Global Consciousness Project in the form of a standard normal deviate (z-scores) for each of 415 formally specified global events from August 1998 to May 2012. For every event, the method of analyzing the data associated with each event is specified before the data are examined. Chance expectation is zero; the grand mean of all the event outcomes is astronomically above chance.

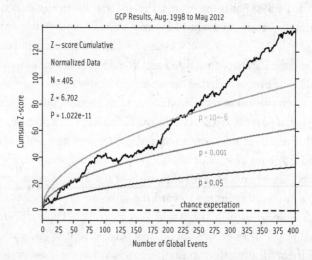

Figure 10. Cumulative deviation from chance expectation is shown as the dashed horizontal line at 0 deviation. Truly random data would produce a curve wavering around that horizontal line. The parabolas show the 0.05 and 0.001 and 0.000001 probability envelopes that indicate significant versus chance deviations. The gradually increasing line shows the statistical results of the Global Consciousness Project from its inception in August 1998 through May 2012.

GCP Results Compared with Random Simulations

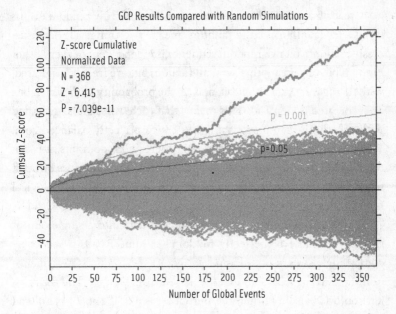

Figure 11. Comparison of actual experimental data as compared to 401 equivalent length but simulated experiments using freshly generated random data.

Exclusive OR

So far we've considered studies involving electronic RNGs. Such devices have been shown to change their statistical behavior in alignment with human intention and attention.[197] Studies using RNGs were originally designed based on a theory developed in the 1970s to explain the underlying physical mechanisms of psi; it was called the "observational theory," or OT.[295]

The fundamental assumption behind OT was simple: "The act of observation by a motivated observer of an event with a quantum mechanically uncertain outcome influences that outcome." This proposal is based on an interpretation of the *quantum measurement problem*, which we will address in more detail soon. It is also why the source of randomness in the original RNGs was based on quantum events.

Creating an RNG that generates sequences of truly random events is not a trivial affair. "Truly random" means two things: (1) Each successive random bit in a random sequence is independent of every other random bit, or said another way, all random bits are freshly generated, with no regard to any other bit; and (2) the probability with which bits are generated is identical. This means that each 0 or 1 bit is generated with exactly the same probability, ½, like a perfectly balanced coin. When you make an electronic circuit to create random bits, it is not too difficult to satisfy criterion (1), but criterion (2) is far more difficult to establish. Thus, to satisfy (2), what is usually done is to add a logical filter to the output of the RNG called an exclusive OR, or XOR.

The XOR logic filter combines random data into a single output that is very close to perfectly random. In some RNGs it works by comparing a stream of random bits against the comparison sequence 010101. . . . If the XOR sees that the first random bit is a 0, and the comparison bit is also a 0, then the output bit is a 0. If one bit is a 1 and the other is a 0, then the output bit is a 1. If both bits are 1s, then the output bit is a 0. Through this process, the average RNG output over the long term will be very close to chance expectation, even if the random data stream catastrophically fails and starts to output only 0s or only 1s.

RNGs employed in the vast majority of psi experiments have used XOR filters, which guarantees that their average behavior will be close to ideal randomness. The results of those tests indicate that *something* interesting is going on, so we have good justification for continuing to study mind-matter interactions.

But attempting to trace the results of those RNG studies backward, like a reverse engineering problem, where we try to understand *why* the randomness changed, is not easy. The XOR logic masks the identity of the original "raw" bits, and in addition the random samples used in these studies are created by summing up a series of random bits, and that summing process also hides what is going on at the level of each individual bit.

These limitations led us to design a new type of micro-PK experiment. To understand what we did, and why the results of the experiments are interesting, requires a little background in the quantum measurement problem.

Quantum Measurement

[The double-slit experiment] has in it the heart of quantum mechanics. In reality, it contains the only mystery.

—*Richard Feynman*[296]

The mystery Feynman was referring to in the preceding quote is the curious fact that a quantum object behaves like a particle when it is observed, but it behaves like a wave when it's not observed. This can be easily demonstrated in a double-slit interferometer, which is a simple device in which one sends particles of light (or electrons, or any elementary particle) through two tiny slits and then records the pattern of light that emerges onto a screen, or a camera.

One might expect that if particles of light (called photons) behaved like separate hunks of stuff, like tiny marbles, then the pattern of light emerging from two slits would always be two bright bands of light. And indeed, if you track each photon as it passes through the slits, then that is what you will see on the screen. However, if you do *not* trace the photons' paths, then you will see an alternating sequence of light and dark bands, called an "interference pattern." This then is the mystery of the dual nature of light—whether you see a wavelike or particle pattern on the screen depends on how you're looking at it. It's as though all matter—photons, electrons, molecules, and so on[297]—"knows" that it is being watched. This exquisitely sensitive bashfulness, known in physics jargon as wave-particle complementarity, lies at the heart of quantum mechanics.

It is also known as the quantum measurement problem, or QMP. It's a problem because it violates the commonsense assumption that we live in an objective reality that is completely independent of observers. The founders of quantum theory, including Neils Bohr, Max Planck, Louis de Broglie, Werner Heisenberg, Erwin Schrödinger, and Albert Einstein, knew that introducing the notion of the observer into quantum theory was a radical change in how physics had been practiced, and they all wrote about the consequences of this change.

A few physicists, like Wolfgang Pauli, Pascual Jordan, and Eugene Wigner, believed that consciousness was not merely important but was fundamentally responsible for the formation of reality. Jordan wrote, "Observations not only disturb what has to be measured, they produce it. . . . We compel [the electron] to assume a definite position. . . . We ourselves produce the results of measurement" (p. 151).[298]

This "strong view" of the role of consciousness in the QMP has been endorsed by renowned physicists ranging from John von Neumann to Bernard d'Espagnat, and later from Euan Squires to Henry Stapp.[299-302] The significance of the proposition and the prominence of those who proposed it makes the idea difficult to blithely ignore, but it challenges a deeply held intuition that the physical world was here, more or less in its present form, long before human consciousness evolved to observe it. As a result, many scientists strongly resist the idea that consciousness could possibly have anything to do with the formation of physical reality.[303-304]

A somewhat softer view of the QMP was expressed by physicist John Bell, who protested that

the concept of "measurement" becomes so fuzzy on reflection that it is quite surprising to have it appearing in physical theory *at the most fundamental level.* . . . [D]oes not any *analysis* of measurement require concepts more *fundamental* than measurement? And should not the fundamental theory be about these more fundamental concepts?[305] (p. 117)

While Bell did not explicitly nominate consciousness for that fundamental concept, it is regarded by some as the core of the measurement process.

One approach to eliminating the observer from the QMP has been to reframe the problem by proposing that all that observation does is increase our knowledge about a measured system. Thus, according to University of Vienna physicist Anton Zeilinger, "The so-called measurement problem . . . is not a problem but a consequence of the more fundamental role information plays in quantum physics as compared to classical physics" (p. 288).[306] Another approach is to argue that "decoherence theory," which argues that quantum effects are washed out through interactions with the environment, eliminates the QMP. But this proposal also has its critics.[307–308] Physicist Jeffrey Bub called decoherence theory an "ignorance interpretation" that does not resolve the QMP.[309]

Others have nonchalantly finessed the QMP by simply denying that there ever was a problem. According to physicist Sheldon Goldstein, "Many physicists pay lip service to . . . the notion that quantum mechanics is about observation or results of measurement. But hardly anybody truly believes this anymore—and it is hard for me to believe anyone really ever did."[303]

Still others propose that the only unambiguous way to avoid the role of the observer in physics is to deny the belief that we have free will.[310] While free will as a persistent brain-generated illusion is a popular idea in the neurosciences today,[171] that idea remains at odds with the only direct form of contact we will ever have with reality—subjective experience—which paradoxically allows for the experience of deciding to believe that free will does not exist.

Philosophical and theoretical arguments aside, the double-slit experiment suggests a novel way to explore the possible role of consciousness in the QMP and a link between a well-accepted (although not well understood) physical phenomenon and a direct relationship between mind and matter.

Two Slits

The double-slit experiment provides in-your-face proof that the world is fundamentally quantum. Thomas Young first described this experiment in 1801, and two centuries later, readers of *Physics World* magazine voted it as "the most beautiful experiment" in physics. As described in the *New York Times*,

> Though [light] is not simply made of particles, neither can it be described purely as a wave. In the first five years of the 20th century, Max Planck and then Albert Einstein showed, respectively, that light is emitted and absorbed in packets—called photons. But other experiments continued to verify that light is also wavelike.
>
> It took quantum theory . . . to reconcile how both ideas could be true: photons and other subatomic particles—electrons, protons, and so forth—exhibit two complementary qualities; they are, as one physicist put it, "wavicles."
>
> To explain the idea . . . physicists often used a thought experiment, in which Young's double-slit demonstration is repeated with a beam of electrons instead of light. Obeying the laws of quantum mechanics, the stream of particles would split in two, and the smaller streams would interfere with each other, leaving the same kind of light- and dark-striped pattern as was cast by light. Particles would act like waves.[311]

In 1961, this idea was actually tested with electrons, and it worked as expected. Elementary particles, chunks of stuff like little billiard balls, behave like waves, *provided that you aren't looking*. This can be demonstrated easily even if you shoot a single photon one at a time through a double-slit apparatus.[312] However—and this is the frosting on the quantum measurement problem—those very same chunks of stuff behave like particles when you *do* look at them. Technically, the process of looking is called gaining "which-path" information, in which you learn which path a photon took as it traveled through the double-slit apparatus.

To repeat: If you *know* that it goes through the left slit or the right slit, typically determined using a detector placed behind each slit, then the photon will behave like a particle. But if you *don't know*, then it will behave like a wave.

Assumptions

The experiment we conducted took advantage of this intriguing effect. It was based on two assumptions:

(A) If information is gained—*by any means*—about a photon's path as it travels through two slits, then the quantum wavelike interference pattern, produced by photons traveling through the slits, will "collapse" in proportion to the certainty of the knowledge obtained.

(B) If some aspect of consciousness is a primordial, self-aware feature of the fabric of reality, and that property is modulated by us through capacities we enjoy as attention and intention, then focusing human attention on a double-slit system may extract information about the photon's path, and in turn that will affect the interference pattern.

The first of these assumptions is very well established.[313] The second, based on the philosophical idea of panpsychism, which we will discuss later, is a controversial but respectable concept within the philosophy of mind.[53]

After reviewing the relevant literature on the measurement problem, physicists Bruce Rosenblum and Fred Kuttner concluded that while most physicists do not believe that observation *literally* creates reality, something about observation remains deeply important and mysterious:

If we assume that no observable physical phenomena exist other than those specified by the present quantum theory, a role for the observer in the experiment can be denied only at the expense of challenging the belief that the observer makes free choices. Therefore no interpretation of the present theory can establish a lack of dependence on the observer to the extent possible in classical physics.[310]

Previous Studies

Because the quantum measurement problem is central to interpretations of quantum theory, philosophical and theoretical discussions about this problem abound in the physics literature. One might expect to find a correspondingly robust experimental literature testing these ideas. But it is not so, and the reason is not mystifying.

That consciousness is linked to the formation of physical reality is associated more with horror movies and medieval magic than it is with sober science. As a result, it is safer for one's scientific career to avoid associating with such dubious topics, and thus it is rare to find such studies reported in the physics literature.

Indeed, the taboo about asking uncomfortable questions is so strong that it even extends to experimental tests of the philosophical foundations of quantum theory, which for more than fifty years was considered untouchable for serious scientists.[314] As noted by historian Olival Freire in discussing the history of tests of Bell's theorem,

> some of the physicists who decided not to hire Clauser [the first to test quantum entanglement] were influenced by the prejudice that experiments on hidden variables were not "real physics." His former adviser, P. Thaddeus, wrote letters warning people not to hire Clauser to do experiments on hidden variables in quantum mechanics as it was "junk science," a view shared by other potential employers.[314] (p. 284)

That this sort of prejudice rears its ugly head even within the pristine rationality of academic physics may be disappointing, but here is where the power of experimental science shines. Unlike most philosophical and religious arguments, which are happily sustained for millennia if given half a chance, science can settle perplexing questions with experiments, or at least it can inform the problem in a new way that might lead to a resolution. That never happens in, say, debates over theological problems.

Four classes of previous psi experiments have studied the quantum measurement problem.[295] They involve (a) studies testing the effects of intention on the statistical behavior of random events linked to quantum sources, as discussed earlier in this chapter;[196, 197, 281, 315, 316] (b) studies involving macroscopic systems such as the use of human physiology as "targets" of intentional influence, as discussed in the last chapter;[2, 194] (c) experiments involving sequential observation to see whether a second observer could consciously or unconsciously detect if a quantum event had been observed by a first observer (which we won't be discussing here);[316–318] and (d) our focus now on experiments investigating conscious influence of photons (particles of light) in optical interferometers.[319–321]

Experiment

Together these four classes of experiments comprise nearly a thousand experiments conducted by over a hundred investigators over six decades.[2] Of these studies, the one that most closely matches Feynman's reference to the "only mystery," as elegantly demonstrated in the double-slit experiment, was a study reported in 1998 by physicists Michael Ibison of Princeton University and Stanley Jeffers of York University.[320]

Jeffers asked a team of participants at York to "'visualize' (observe, by extra-sensory means) monochromatic light passing through a double slit, prior to its registration as an interference pattern by an optical detector" (p. 543).[320] Ibison asked a team at Princeton, using an improved apparatus, to mentally intend that a bar graph indicating the contrast between optical interference patterns recorded with and without observation "to remain as low as possible" (p. 546).[320] In other words, they monitored aspects of the double-slit interference patterns while people were observing the system with their mind's eye alone, and recording if the interference patterns changed in predictable ways. Did the particles of light "know" that they were being watched, even when the watcher was just the human mind?

In both cases the mental effort periods were thirty seconds in length, and these were alternated with no-effort control periods. The team at Princeton reported marginally significant experimental evidence in favor of an observational effect, and the team at York reported a nonsignificant result (although curiously their data showed a significantly larger sample variance than would be expected by chance, suggesting that there might have been an effect, but it was not stable from one participant to the next).

In interpreting this ambivalent outcome it is useful to know that the Princeton test employed a small team of dedicated participants who were experienced with maintaining focused intention in these types of experiments, and the test was conducted in a laboratory where the staff was sympathetic to the possibility of mind-matter interactions. By contrast, the York test employed unselected participants recruited without regard to their interest or skill in the task, and by an experimenter who was curious but not experienced in conducting tasks with human participants.

Michelson Interferometer

We decided to repeat this experiment first using a Michelson interferometer rather than a double-slit apparatus.[322] All optical interferometers exhibit the same basic effect, that is, wavelike interference patterns when the observer doesn't know how the photons traveled through the optical apparatus, and particle-like diffraction patterns when the observer does know.

The Michelson interferometer consists of two "arms," each several inches in length, as shown in Figure 12. One of those arms was the target area, where we asked people to imagine that they could see, with their mind's eye alone, the photons as they traveled in that area. If their imagination actually perceived the photons (via clairvoyance, given that this task did not involve the ordinary senses), then they would hypothetically gain which-path information and cause the wavelike interference to "collapse." The collapse would be in proportion to the degree of information they obtained. Because clairvoyance is rather weak in most people, the amount of collapse that we expected to measure in this experiment was very small.

We used a low power laser to send a one-millimeter beam into the interferometer. The beam passed through a filter to cut down on the illumination intensity, and then it went through a lens and a half-silvered mirror. That mirror caused half the beam to go to one fully reflective mirror and the other half to a second fully reflective mirror.

The two beams reflected off those mirrors were directed back through the half-silvered mirror and then combined into a single beam to create an interference pattern. That pattern was recorded by a highly sensitive, thermoelectrically cooled digital camera, which was controlled by a computer to record digital images at a rate of one per second.

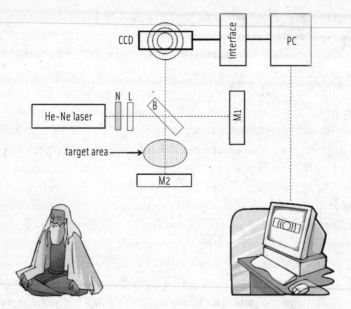

Figure 12. A low power Helium-Neon laser was reduced in intensity by passing it through a neutral density filter (N), the resulting beam was directed through a diverging lens (L), then a half-silvered beam splitter (B), and then it bounced off two mirrors (M1, M2). The resulting interference pattern passed through a high performance narrow-band notch filter and was imaged onto a thermoelectricly cooled digital camera (CCD). The optical system was housed inside a vibration, acoustic, and electromagnetically shielded, double-steel-walled room. During experimental sessions, the shielded chamber was light-tight, and the computer controlling the camera was remotely controlled by a second computer outside the chamber via a fiber-optic connection. Participants sat quietly outside the shielded chamber.

Optical interferometers are incredibly sensitive. Tiny vibrations in the ground caused by trucks driving a half mile away can smear the interference pattern if the interferometer is not heavily isolated from the environment. Our apparatus was secured to the floor of a twenty-eight-hundred-pound, double-steel-walled, electromagnetically shielded, optically sealed room, which in turn rested on a vibration isolation mat on a ground-level concrete floor.

During a test session, participants sat quietly, one at a time, on a chair or on the floor, about six feet from the outer wall of the shielded chamber. I asked each participant to imagine that he or she could mentally "see" the photons in the target arm of the interferometer. Or, if they found this too difficult to imagine, they could try to mentally "block" the photons. They did this with eyes closed, sitting quietly outside the shielded room.

The computer automatically took camera shots of the interference pattern, and I announced each test run condition following a preset sequence of counterbalanced conditions: *concentrate* on the interferometer now, or *relax* and withdraw your attention from the interferometer.

Analysis

Each experimental session consisted of a series of concentrate and relax periods, each lasting twenty-five seconds and alternating for a total of seven minutes. This may not sound particularly taxing, but to do this task with high concentration and stable focus is much more difficult than it seems. Without meditation practice, thoughts begin to wander every couple of seconds, so even in sessions lasting just a few minutes, most nonmeditators' minds begin to drift into mouthwatering fantasies about cheeseburgers rather than the experiment under way. To see if the ability to focus attention was a factor in the outcome of this experiment, some of the participants recruited for this study were required to have experience in one or more mental focusing techniques, such as meditation.

Figure 13 (top) shows an interference pattern as captured in one frame of the camera when both arms of the interferometer were open (i.e., both split beams were allowed to pass through the interferometer unobstructed). The variations in the plot indicate the image intensity recorded at different locations. Figure 13 (bottom) shows what happens when I blocked the "mental target area" in one of the interferometer arms with a piece of opaque plastic. These images show only a tiny portion of the interference pattern because the camera aperture was rather small.

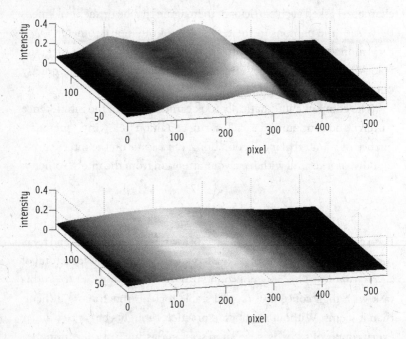

Figure 13. Images recorded by the digital camera in a half-second exposure. The top image shows the illumination intensity (z axis) observed when both arms of the interferometer were open; the bottom image shows the intensity pattern when one arm of the interferometer was physically blocked.

From these images we can see that blocking one arm of the interferometer caused two conspicuous changes: The wavy interference pattern transformed into a flatter pattern and the overall level of light intensity dropped. The former occurred because the wavelike interference pattern was eliminated by blocking one of the light beams. The latter effect occurred because about half the available photons were prevented from reaching the camera.

Then I calculated the average illumination level collapsed across the y-axis in Figure 14; this resulted in a curve providing an average cross section of illumination. If we now take the grand average across fifty of these cross-section images, captured by the camera one second apart in both the blocked and open conditions, we obtain the two curves shown in Figure 14 and the difference between them in Figure 15.

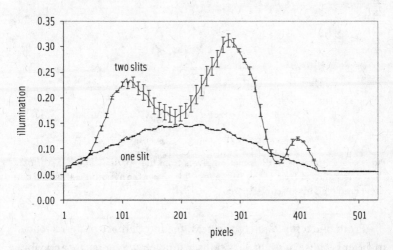

Figure 14. Average illumination intensity in the passed (both slits open) and blocked (one slit closed) conditions, based on fifty frames in each condition. Standard deviation error bars are shown for both curves. For the one-slit condition the error bars are quite small, indicating the stability of the laser and camera. The larger error bars in the two-slit condition reflect the exquisite sensitivity of the interferometer to environmental fluctuations.

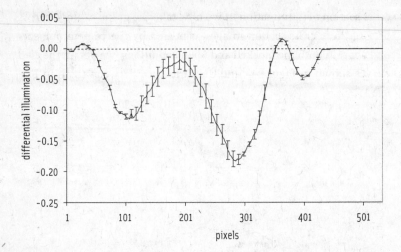

Figure 15. Difference in illumination levels from the previous figure. Error bars show one standard error of the difference. This shows the hypothetically ideal outcome predicted in this experiment.

From one test session to the next, the interference patterns tended to differ because of slight variations in ambient temperature and vibration. So for the sake of simplicity I based the formal statistical analysis not on a change in the precise shape of the interference pattern, but rather on a decrease in the average illumination level over the entire camera image during the concentration or "mental blocking" condition as compared to the relaxed or "mental passing" condition.

To test the design and analytical procedures for possible problems, I also included control runs to allow the system to record interference patterns automatically without anyone being present in the laboratory or paying attention to the interferometer. Data from those control sessions were analyzed in the same way as in the experimental sessions.

Results

I was fortunate to recruit five meditators, four of whom had many decades of daily meditative practice. Those five contributed nine test sessions. Five other individuals with no meditation experience, or less than two years of practice, contributed nine additional sessions. I referred to the latter group as nonmeditators.

I predicted an overall negative score for each experimental session (illustrated by the idealized negative curve shown in Figure 15). The combined results were in fact significantly negative, with odds against chance of 500 to 1. The identical analysis across all the control sessions resulted in odds against chance of close to 1 to 1, indicating that the experimental results were not due to procedural or analytical biases.

Figure 16 shows the cumulative score (in terms of standard normal deviates, or z-scores) for the nine sessions contributed by experienced meditators and nine other sessions involving nonmeditators. The experienced meditators resulted in a combined odds against chance of 107,000 to 1, and the nonmeditators obtained results close to chance expectation. This supported my conjecture that meditators would be better at this task than nonmeditators.

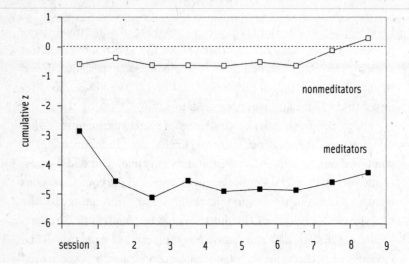

Figure 16. Experienced meditators (more than two years of daily practice) obtained combined odds against chance of 107,000 to 1. Nonmeditators obtained results close to chance.

Something Strange

The experimental session contributed by the most experienced meditator was especially interesting. The bold curve in Figure 17 shows the difference between the concentration versus relaxed conditions for that experimental session, and the thin curve shows the exact same analysis applied to a control session run immediately afterward, in which no one was present.

From these curves we can see that the *magnitude* of the change in illumination was minuscule, but the error bars show that the concentration versus relaxed difference in the experimental data was downward, as predicted, and far from a chance effect, which would be a flat line in this analysis. By contrast, in the control session the difference was indeed flat. The error bars in both sessions were about the same, indicating that the results of the experimental session were not due to unexpected movements.

It's important to realize that the curve in Figure 17 was produced by a meditator sitting quietly outside the sealed chamber that contained the interferometer. This outcome, which closely resembles what would happen if you physically blocked a laser beam with your hand, was caused (it appears) by the meditator's *mind* alone.

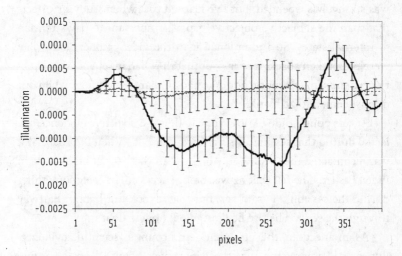

Figure 17. Average illumination levels for experimental (bold, bottom line) and control (thin, top line) sessions, with standard error bars. Note that the error bars in both cases are about the same, indicating that the lower illumination level recorded during the experimental run was not due to artifacts.

This session showed intriguing objective evidence for a mind-matter interaction effect, but an unusual subjective event also happened that is worth mentioning. For this session, knowing that the planned participant was a highly experienced meditator, I decided to have it filmed for future reference. I asked two videographers to shoot the session as it unfolded. They set up their cameras and started filming, the meditator prepared himself mentally for about ten minutes, then signaled that he was ready to begin.

I started the experiment and it proceeded without incident until about halfway through the session. Then for a few seconds I felt strangely disoriented, as though all my mental activity suddenly stopped. I shook off this odd sensation, and the disorientation soon passed. The session ended, I thanked the meditator, and he left. Then I spent a few minutes discussing the session with the two videographers as they gathered up their gear.

I didn't attribute much meaning to that moment when my mind was strangely suspended, but I've learned that when studying effects that span the subjective-objective gap, it's important to pay attention to internal states. So I mentioned it to the videographers, and they were both taken aback. It turns out that they had independently experienced the same phenomenon. We had all shared a moment when our minds seemed to go blank.

At this point I didn't know yet whether the objective evidence collected during that session was significant or not. When I found that it was, I contacted the meditator, who by then was back at his ashram in India. I asked if he felt that he was being successful in *doing* something during the session. He said yes, but that it took until about halfway through the session before he figured out how to do it.

As an anecdote, this episode doesn't count as scientific evidence. But it's still interesting that the experiment obtained objective evidence of a mind-matter interaction effect at precisely the same time that three people unexpectedly felt something strange occur.

The Michelson interferometer experiment suggested that an observed optical system does behave differently than an unobserved system, and in a way that's suggestive of the quantum observer effect. In other words, we—like others before us—had once again found evidence for a direct mind-matter interaction. This was interesting, but it wasn't enough. What we wanted to know was whether mind-matter interaction effects were consistent with the notion that consciousness "collapses" the quantum wave function. If it turned out that this was the case, then the most successful physical theory in history might contain the seeds of psychokinesis within it.

Double-Slit Experiment

We decided to follow up the Michelson interferometer study using an optical double-slit system.[323] The apparatus we designed directed a low-power laser beam through a filter to further reduce the illumination intensity, and then through two slits etched into a metal foil slide. Each slit was 10 microns (millionths of a meter) wide, and they were separated by a space of 200 microns. The wavelike interference pattern produced by this apparatus was recorded by a high-resolution digital camera (3,000 pixels, all in a line), and the whole apparatus was housed inside a custom-machined, light-tight aluminum box.

To test if observation by the mind's eye changes the interference pattern, one approach would be to keep track of the maximum illumination level (called a "peak") around pixel 1500 in Figure 18-A, and also of the minimum illumination levels (called "troughs") around 60 pixels before and after the peak. If the wavelike nature of light "collapsed" due to observation, then the peak would drop (a little) and the troughs would rise (a lot). These were the measurements of interest to Stanley Jeffers and Michael Ibison when they did their test with a double-slit system.

We decided to use a more general method. We were interested not in how specific peaks or troughs were behaving, but in how the entire interference pattern changed when people were asked to direct their attention toward or away from it.

This involved calculating a spectral or Fourier transform of the interference pattern image captured by the camera. This is less complex than it may sound. It's analogous to determining the frequency spectrum of an audio signal. For example, Figure 18-A shows a snapshot of the double-slit interference pattern as it was imaged onto the camera. The wavy pattern shows light intensity—the brighter the light, the higher the graph.

If you can imagine that this wasn't a camera image but rather part of an audio signal, then you can see that the pattern consists of two main frequencies: a faster-moving frequency associated with the interference produced by light passing through a double slit, and a slower-moving frequency associated with the diffraction pattern produced by each of the two individual slits (i.e., the bell-like shape that constrains the faster frequencies).

The Fourier transform of the pattern in Figure 18-A is shown in Figure 18-B. Three spectral peaks are clearly evident. The peak near the value 1 on the x-axis represents a slower-moving frequency associated with each of the single slits (call this S), and the peak at 45 presents the faster-moving frequency associated with the two slits acting together as a double slit (call this D). The peak at 90 is a resonance (called a "harmonic") of the one at 45. The ratio of the double to single spectral peaks, which we will refer to as the power ratio R, where $R = D / S$, was the variable we used to measure how much "double-slit-iness" there was in the interference pattern over the course of the experiment.

During a test session, a participant—let's call her Daisy—was instructed by a computer-synthesized voice to concentrate her attention toward the double-slit apparatus or to withdraw her attention and relax. When asked to concentrate, Daisy directed her attention toward the two tiny slits located inside the double-slit optical system. It was explained that this task was purely in the "mind's eye," that is, an act of imagination.

To some people this instruction proved to be too abstract, so to assist their imaginations they were shown a five-minute cartoon animation of the double-slit experiment, where a particle detector was portrayed as being analogous to a human eye. If the task was still unclear, we suggested that Daisy try to mentally block one of the slits, or to "become one with" the optical system in a contemplative way, or to mentally push the laser beam to cause it to go through one of the two slits rather than both.

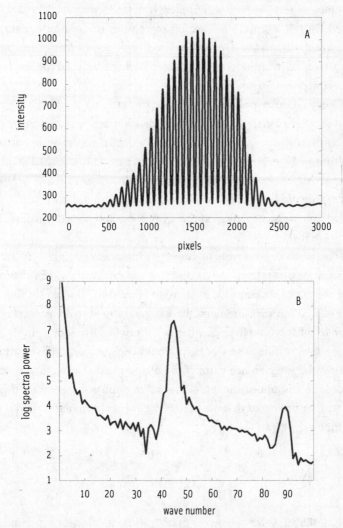

Figure 18 (A). Interference pattern intensity recorded in a double-slit optical system by a 3,000-pixel line camera, averaged over ten thousand camera frames. This pattern shows how light behaves like interfering waves (similar to waves in water) as long as you don't know the path each photon takes when it goes through the slits. Figure 18 (B). Log of spatial spectral power with double-slit power peaking around spectral wave number 45 and single-slit power at 1. The peak around wave number 90 is the first harmonic of the double-slit frequency.

Once a test session was under way, the computer's voice directed Daisy's attention toward or away from the optical system in fifteen-second periods. One test session consisted of forty such periods presented in a randomized counterbalanced order of concentrate-relax-concentrate-relax, and so on.

Daisy sat quietly about two meters from the sealed double-slit apparatus. She wasn't allowed to touch or approach it at any time. All the sessions were conducted inside our shielded test chamber at the Institute of Noetic Sciences. This chamber in its unadorned state is a rather imposing steel cube without windows, so to make it more welcoming we covered the walls and ceiling with a muslin fabric, installed antistatic carpeting on the steel floor, and placed comfortable furniture inside.

The predicted outcome of this experiment was straightforward: If consciousness is related to "collapse" of the quantum wave function, then the act of concentrating attention toward the double slit should have caused our measurement, the spectral ratio R, to *decrease* as compared to what would happen when withdrawing attention. This is because the wavelike aspect of light would decline due to observation, causing the interference pattern to collapse, and that in turn would reduce the amount of "double-slit-iness" or double-slit spectral power. We further predicted that meditators would perform better than non-meditators.

Results

EXPERIMENT 1. Over a two-year period, we conducted six experiments with the double-slit system. In the first pilot study we found that the spectral ratio R did decline modestly in accordance with the "collapse" hypothesis, with odds of 17 to 1. Meditators performed slightly better, with odds of 18 to 1, and nonmeditators obtained results near chance. Control tests using the same equipment in the same location, but without participants present, also showed a nonsignificant result. The effect size for all experimental sessions combined was $es = -0.26$ (we predicted a decline, so a negative effect size is in the expected direction), which as we've seen is close to the magnitude of the average effect size observed across tens of thousands of behavioral and social sciences studies, and also similar to studies often observed in psi experiments.

EXPERIMENT 2. In the second experiment, we developed a way to provide real-time audio feedback of the R signal, and we increased the attention epoch lengths to thirty seconds. For feedback, during relaxed periods the computer played a soft droning tone, and during concentration periods it played a musical note that changed pitch to reflect the up or down movement of the R signal. Participants were told that if they were successful during the concentration periods, then the pitch of the musical note would go *down* (to indicate collapse of the wave function).

This study again provided evidence in favor of the hypothesis, with modest odds against chance of 12 of 1. Again the meditators showed better performance with odds against chance of 48 to 1; non-meditators' results were close to chance. In terms of effect size, this experiment showed overall results that were nearly identical to the first experiment, with $es = -0.25$.

EXPERIMENT 3. In the third study, we explored if the proximity of the participants near the optical system might have influenced the interference pattern. While heat differences associated with small changes in body position six and a half feet away from the optical system would amount to temperature changes of a tiny fraction of a degree, we still wanted to check if the optical system systematically expanded or contracted slightly due to potential temperature fluctuations.

To do this, we placed four sensitive thermocouples on the optical system and in front of it. Then we had thirteen people conduct thirty-three test sessions, and we identified all the test sessions that showed a marked drop in R. For those sessions we investigated whether the thermocouple measurements also showed a change in temperature. If they did, then what we had previously observed might have been due to changes in ambient temperature rather than to shifts in attention.

Six meditators contributed 22 sessions and 7 nonmeditators contributed 11 sessions. The 22 meditator sessions resulted in an effect size comparable to the effect produced by meditators in the first experiment ($es = -0.39$ vs. -0.32, respectively). To then test for temperature-mediated effects, we examined all the sessions contributed by meditators that resulted in negative scores. There were 16 such sessions. Remember, "negative" in this study means effects going in the predicted direction.

Results of that analysis found no significant temperature differences, not on the laser tube itself, the double-slit apparatus housing, or in front of the apparatus, or within a meter in front of the participant. This told us that the robust decline in R observed in the 16 selected sessions was not driven by systematic variations in temperature. So proximity of the human body did not explain the results we were seeing.

EXPERIMENT 4. In our fourth experiment, we tested a "nonlocal" aspect of the consciousness collapse interpretation. This is a bit tricky to grasp at first, because it invokes the timeless nature of the quantum world. I'll go through this slowly.

The idea that the quantum wave function collapses due to observation implies that the collapse occurs only when observation occurs, *and not when the data are generated*.[295] That is, unlike events in the everyday world, where actions occur in particular locations and unfold in ordinary clock time, events in the quantum domain do not occur *in time* as we normally experience it. This is what is meant by the spooky "nonlocal" nature of quantum mechanics—events are connected across the usual limitations of space *and time*.

When an elementary quantum object is not being observed, it remains in what's called an "indeterminate state." In that unobserved condition, the object *has no definite properties* yet—no size, shape, location, polarization, spin, or any other property that we ascribe to ordinary real objects. The consciousness collapse idea further proposes that when, and only when, an object is *consciously* observed does it take on real properties.

To repeat—because this concept may make your brain hurt the first time you encounter it—if you take measurements of a quantum system using an inanimate recording device, like a camera, then that system will remain in an indeterminate state *until it is observed*. This ridiculous-sounding idea has been tested in conventional physics labs and it has definitely been shown to exist. That type of study is called the delayed-choice experiment.[154, 324]

We tested this idea in the present context by using a time-reversed version of our double-slit experiment, somewhat like the studies that Daryl Bem conducted, as discussed earlier in the chapter on precognition. This test also provided a more rigorous way for us to test the effect of participants being located within a few meters of the optical system, because all the data in this study were generated and recorded with the apparatus located by itself inside the shielded chamber, and with no one else present in the laboratory.

To prepare for this study, we recorded fifty sessions in the laboratory in April 2009. No one was present during the data generation and recording process, and the data remained unobserved. In June 2009, participants were asked to view a strip-chart display, which unbeknownst to them was playing back the unobserved data that was recorded in April.

As in the other experiments, they were invited to mentally cause the value *R* to go as low as possible when the computer gave them the instruction to concentrate on the double slit, and to withdraw their attention when given the instruction to relax. The design feature that made this a time-reversed, or retrocausal, experiment was that the attention condition assignments were generated and assigned during the observation phase, which took place three months *after* the data were generated and recorded.

Twenty-two participants were recruited at a conference in Tucson,

Arizona. The test was conducted in an office at the conference hotel. After they completed all their test sessions, 22 of the remaining unobserved data files were used as control sessions. Of the 22 participants, 10 indicated that they had a regular meditation practice; the remaining 12 were classified as nonmeditators. The meditator subgroup supported the hypothesis with odds against chance of 175 to 1. The nonmeditators got chance results.

To emphasize, this suggests that the observational effect is not limited to working in real time; it also works in what, from a conventional point of view, would appear to be *backward* in time. Based on the experimental evidence reviewed in earlier chapters, by now you should be used to the idea that the mind has access to information from "outside" the usual boundaries of space and time. This implies either that the mind can reach *through* space and time, or—and I'm guessing that this is more likely—the mind is not *in* ordinary spacetime in the first place.

While you're contemplating this, I will summarize what we've seen so far. Across the first four double-slit studies we recorded 121 test sessions. All sessions combined resulted in odds against chance of 67 to 1. All 67 meditator sessions resulted in odds against chance of 13,800 to 1, and all 41 nonmeditator sessions resulted in chance. The 149 control sessions produced results uniformly at chance.

EXPERIMENT 5. Our fifth study was designed to formally replicate what we had seen in the first four experiments, with 50 preplanned sessions. We selected 31 participants who we predicted would do well because of their meditation or other attention-focusing practice. The results were remarkable; overall the odds against chance for this were 268,000 to 1. The control sessions showed chance results.

EXPERIMENT 6. In this study we examined the role of participants' personalities and beliefs. We again ran a series of 50 preplanned sessions with 50 participants who, unlike the previous study, where we tried to optimize our selection of people, were recruited volunteers with a broad range of personality traits, meditation experience, and beliefs. Each person filled out a questionnaire asking about their belief in psychic phenomena and their years of meditation or other attention training experiences, and then they filled out a questionnaire to assess the degree to which they can become absorbed in a task while focusing.[325] We asked the question about belief because as previously mentioned, it's been known since the 1940s that openness to the possibility of ESP is a reliable predictor of performance in this type of task.[326]

The overall result in this study was odds against chance of a modest 9 to 1. This smaller magnitude effect size was expected because we had recruited people with a wide range of prior beliefs, meditative experience, and absorption. The fifty control runs were in accordance with chance. We also found that the correlation between performance and belief in psychic phenomena was significant and in the predicted direction, with odds against chance of 30 to 1. The correlations between performance and absorption, and performance and meditation experience, were not statistically significant, possibly because the people we recruited for this study showed a limited range of values for these factors.

Summary of the Double-Slit Experiments

In a series of six experiments testing a "wave function collapse" hypothesis with a double-slit system, we obtained a combined outcome with odds against chance of 184,000 to 1. Control sessions provided no evidence of procedural or analytical artifacts that might have been responsible for these effects. We published these results in the journal *Physics Essays* in 2012.[323] Overall meditators performed better than nonmeditators, with odds against chance of 300,000 to 1. When the results of the meditators' sessions in the Michelson interferometer study are combined with the meditators' data in the double-slit studies, the overall odds against chance accumulate to 3.7 billion to 1. The bottom line—mind and matter interact.

Summary

The scientifically credible evidence for mind-matter interactions is not the in-your-face big effects that stage magicians are fond of debunking. Rather, it's made up of smaller-scale effects that make a certain sense from the perspective of quantum theory. About those micro-PK effects, Patanjali might have said, "Of course mind interacts with matter. Haven't you read the *Yoga Sutras*?" About the macro-PK effects reported in yogic lore and in numerous historical anecdotes, Patanjali might have said, with a hint of annoyance, "Well, there are a few rare yogis who can perform the big effects, but as you know they're cautioned not to display them publicly. Why not focus on the elementary siddhis, like clairvoyance? Those are easy to demonstrate."

CHAPTER 13

Clairvoyance

I was a peripheral visionary. I could see the future, but only way off to the side.

—*Steven Wright*

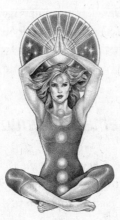

The word *clairvoyance*, from the French, literally means "clear seeing," but the perceptions can resemble sound, called *clairaudience*, or perception of smell, touch, or taste, called *clairsentience*. The term "extra-sensory perception" (ESP) is synonymous with clairvoyance, as are modern euphemisms such as remote viewing, remote perception, and anomalous cognition.

Clairvoyance differs from telepathy in that the information obtained is not "sent" by anyone. It appears to differ from precognition in that the information obtained through clairvoyance is about events at a distance in space, rather than events at a distance in time. And because of the relativity of space and time, if precognition exists then it is likely that clairvoyance also exists.

In previous books, *The Conscious Universe* and *Entangled Minds*, I described a century's worth of scientific experiments investigating various aspects of clairvoyance.[1, 2] The two primary classes of experiments have been forced-choice card guessing tests and free-response picture drawing tests. As with telepathy, precognition, and psychokinesis, the experimental evidence for clairvoyance is abundantly clear—it exists far beyond any reasonable scientific doubt. Patanjali was correct about this class of siddhis—the basic phenomenon exists. But in the *Yoga Sutras*, several types of clairvoyance are described, including some that are quite remarkable.

Extreme Clairvoyance

For example, *Pada* III.26, *Knowledge of the outer universe*, could be interpreted as the ability to perceive at cosmic distances, meaning beyond the earth, to other planets and even to distant star systems. And *Pada* III.27–28, *Knowledge of the inner universe*, suggests that one can perceive microscopic objects, down to elementary particles and possibly smaller.

In one sense these extremes of clairvoyance should not be too surprising, because if one can perceive what's happening in the next room, or in a hidden envelope directly in front of you, then in principle gazing at a planet at the other side of the universe, or watching what's happening inside an atom, should also be possible. That is, clairvoyance is not constrained by ordinary space-time or by the ordinary senses, so what is possible to perceive may be limited more by our imagination than by any absolute measurement of space or time. Fortunately, we don't have to rely only on our imaginations because there is some evidence in support of the more extreme forms of clairvoyance.

The first case involves the artist Ingo Swann, who was instrumental in developing clairvoyance training systems for the US government as part of the research program now popularly known by one of its code names, "Stargate." This formerly top secret project, funded by several Department of Defense and intelligence agencies for over twenty years, was charged with investigating methods to improve the use of clairvoyance for psychic spying. Numerous books are available that describe the aims and findings of Stargate, which included both an active-duty army unit and a civilian research unit.[327–329]

Swann was asked during an early phase of that program, in 1973, to psychically explore the planet Jupiter. The *Pioneer 10* spacecraft was headed toward Jupiter at the time, but there were no close-up photographs so this would provide a good test for the reach of clairvoyance. In Swann's description of Jupiter, on April 27, 1973, he said:

> Very high in the atmosphere there are crystals . . . they glitter. Maybe the stripes are like bands of crystals, maybe like rings of Saturn, though not far out like that. Very close within the atmosphere. I bet you they'll reflect radio probes.[329] (p. 32)

Remember that at the time, there was no evidence at all for rings around Jupiter. There weren't even any reasons to suspect it. Six years later, rings were discovered by the *Voyager* spacecraft. As reported in *Time* magazine,

> and, most surprising of all, [*Voyager*] revealed the presence of a thin, flat ring around the great planet. Said University of

Arizona astronomer Bradford Smith: "We're standing here with our mouths open, reluctant to tear ourselves away."[329] (p. 32)

As for perceiving at the atomic scale, the Theosophists Charles Leadbeater and Annie Besant published their clairvoyant investigations of atomic structure in 1895 in an article entitled "Occult Chemistry" in the Theosophical journal, *Lucifer*. They later expanded their efforts into a book-length treatment, also entitled *Occult Chemistry*. Their studies were for the most part forgotten until physicist Stephen Phillips published a book in 1980, *Extra-Sensory Perception of Quarks*.[330] After reviewing subsequent refinements in his analysis, Phillips concluded in a 1995 publication:

> A century-old claim by two early leaders of the Theosophical Society to have used a form of ESP to observe subatomic particles is evaluated. Their observations are found to be consistent with facts of nuclear physics and with the quark model of particle physics provided that their assumption that they saw atoms is rejected. Their account of the force binding together the fundamental constituents of matter is shown to agree with the string model. Their description of these basic particles bears striking similarity to basic ideas of superstring theory.[331] (p. 489)

These two cases of what we might call macro and micro clairvoyance are intriguing and consistent with *Yoga Sutras, Pada* III.26–28, but there's a subtlety in how we should interpret them. One interpretation is that through clairvoyance it is possible to see, right now, what is happening at the other side of the universe or in the subatomic realm. A second interpretation is that what appears to be clairvoyance is actually more mundane versions of precognition or telepathy, or some mixture of the two. That's because psi perceptions are not limited by present space-time constraints. So if anyone in the future knows about the target of interest, then what appears to be clairvoyance "up" into outer space, or "down" into the atomic realm, might be due to some other, more generalized form of psi perception.

A third interpretation is that both cases were just lucky guesses. That is, there's a big difference between individual case studies and a series of controlled experiments. The former may be intriguing, but the latter provide a known degree of confidence in whether the effects are chance or beyond chance. In this instance, the case studies look good, but we don't know for sure.

And even when there are sound reasons to accept evidence for genuine psi effects, the dilemma of multiple interpretations highlights the epistemological challenges faced when studying phenomena that transcend the usual boundaries of space and time. This problem has led an increasing number of psi researchers to propose that there are basically just two kinds of psi phenomena: an *inflow of information* that we label psi perception, which includes clairvoyance, precognition, and telepathy, and an *outflow of information*, which includes psychokinesis and distant healing. From this perspective, there is really just one underlying phenomenon: Reality itself is constructed from information. We'll discuss this idea in more detail later.

Remote Viewing Example

Rather than repeat the overview of precognitive remote viewing studies mentioned in Chapter 9 (there they were called free-response studies, emphasizing the methodological design), I'll provide a concrete example. Many examples of remote viewing experiments can be found in other books.[327, 329, 332–335]

The case in point involves a professor, Robert Hogan, who taught writing at Illinois State University, the University of Pittsburgh, and other schools. He offered to demonstrate his skill at remote viewing, with him located in Illinois and me in California. I set about finding a small object for Hogan to describe while no one else was in my office, and I told no one that I was going to conduct this test. While searching for a suitable object I glanced at the miniblinds in my office window to see if someone might be able to peek in. The blinds were angled to let light in from above, and there were no tall buildings around, so no one could have seen the object that I ultimately selected and placed into a desk drawer.

The next day I received the following e-mail from Hogan:

As usual, I have more than one distinct impression. I'll describe one at a time.

The first that came through is like a dark gold, rounded, lined or burnished texture, narrowing as it goes upwards to a round top. Shiny, felt like metal but could be wood or ceramic.

Second was green to yellow green, impression of flying at treetop level, something large going through the green, motion, large mass.

Third was gold, red, bronzy, with smaller, round, sculpted smooth parts, like a figure, but the parts are deeply sculpted.

The object I had selected was a bronze-colored, plastic Northwest Airlines pin, which I had taped to a yellow-green Post-it note. I selected this item because it is not something one would ordinarily expect to find in an office environment.

I asked Hogan to describe his process in performing this task. He replied:

In 1998, I read *Tracks in the Psychic Wilderness* by Dale Graff[333] [retired Defense Intelligence Agency director of the US government's classified psi research program] in which he described how to remote view. I sat in front of a monitor with the code for a target in my mind and closed my eyes. I made my mind "an empty rice bowl." I repeated the code to myself and waited. The impressions came and I sketched them. I nailed the target the first time.

What I do hasn't changed much [since then], but I have some nuances that are different. I go to a quiet place and sit. I close my eyes and warm down for a minute or two by relaxing. [Former army "psychic spy"] Joe McMoneagle takes 45 minutes to warm down. I'd be asleep by then. I can go only a minute or two. With my eyes closed, I blank my mind and repeat the target code or location. It could be a code like [the letters] AMEF or a location like "on the table in Wayne's office." I just need something to focus my attention on that thing out of the innumerable other things in the universe. I have a place I "look" in my mind, and I know my eyes actually focus on it. It isn't like an infinity setting on a camera. I think it's with a focus of about three feet.

The next part is difficult to describe. I allow images to come. If someone says it's an object on a table, I allow an "impression" of a table to come into that space. I'm not really remote viewing the table. It's just a platform. Then my mind relaxes into allowing target impressions through. I may say, "Let me see the object on Wayne's table." As I relax into it, I get a feeling that is a little like a very small feeling of that time when you're starting to drift into sleep.

I could guess it's going from Alpha [brainwave rhythm] into Theta, but I don't know. I don't hold it for long, though. I come back from it and have to go back in. I have to open my eyes and sketch what I get, but I'm not a good artist and by the time I get a part of a sketch started, I've lost some of the target. I write the impressions in words and sketch what I can. Then I have to close my eyes again, warm down briefly, and repeat the process. I have to stay with details and avoid naming something. I'm much better at objects than pictures.

I've learned that everything I get is meaningful, but some

can't be associated with an object. It's still attached to some real thing. I have had no training, and probably haven't done more than a hundred sessions since I first learned I could do it in 1998.

As I was preparing this chapter, it occurred to me to ask Hogan where he was living when he performed this test. His reply: "Normal, Illinois." Patanjali would have laughed.

Robert Hogan spends just a few minutes meditating, he had no formal training in clairvoyance, and he hardly ever practices. And yet he is able to accurately perceive a target thousands of miles away. Perhaps he is naturally gifted with the siddhi of clairvoyance, which Patanjali mentions is one way that the siddhis can manifest.

But the *Yoga Sutras* also tell us that the development of the siddhis is intimately related to yoga practice, and in particular to the meditation component of yoga. Is there any scientific evidence supporting this claim? We've already seen in the studies involving mind-matter interaction with optical interferometers that meditators performed better than nonmeditators, and we saw a similar outcome in the precognition study testing brain activity in meditators and nonmeditators. Have any other studies found this same trend?

Summary

The historical, anecdotal, case study and scientific evidence for clairvoyance is consistent—this ability is real. The only aspect that might have surprised Patanjali is that a future civilization would arise in which some would declare clairvoyance to be impossible on theoretical grounds. Then again, perhaps he did foresee this, but he also knew that scientific theories come and go, and that a more sophisticated model of reality would develop in the fullness of time that would acknowledge clairvoyance as a subset of something even more remarkable.

CHAPTER 14

Psi and Meditation

"Students achieving Oneness will move on to Twoness.

—*Woody Allen*

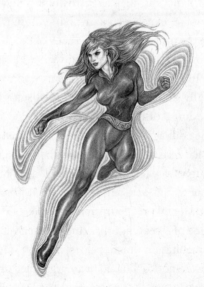

As interest in meditation was rising on the popular front in the 1970s, researchers began to study the relationship between psi and meditation. Many of those studies explicitly acknowledged Patanjali's prescription for developing the siddhis and were aimed at testing if those claims could be verified in the laboratory.

One of the first studies of this type was reported by psychologist Gertrude Schmeidler in 1970.[336] She tested six graduate students in psychology having little knowledge or interest in either psi or meditation. They performed a simple forced-choice ESP test before and after instruction of meditation and breathing techniques (pranayama) by an Indian yogi. Performance before meditation was at chance; afterward it was significantly above chance.

Other experiments reported in the 1970s and 1980s involved one of three designs: (1) participants who meditated before and after a forced-choice or free-response clairvoyance test; (2) meditators versus non-meditators in psychokinetic tasks; and (3) studies of brain electrical activity in meditators to see if certain brain states were associated with improved performance during a telepathy test.

A summary of 16 experiments involving these three designs performed through the mid-1970s showed that 9 of the 16 reported experiments were statistically significant, each with odds against chance of at least 20 to 1. In a group of 16 experiments one would expect only one study (actually slightly less than one) to be statistically significant by chance. So finding 9 of 16 studies reported as significant is most unlikely; in fact, the odds against chance are 61 million to 1.[168] Schmeidler later reviewed that research literature and then expanded it to studies completed through 1994. She modestly concluded "Meditation is conducive to ESP success if (and only if) the meditators wholeheartedly accept the experimental procedure and the goals of the research."[337]

This early line of research, consisting of just over a dozen studies, suggested that meditation practice does seem to improve psi ability, but the studies were not conducted in an organized or long-term manner, and so the conclusion at the time remained tentative.[338]

Interest in the meditation-psi relationship began to decline as the ganzfeld telepathy experiments became popular, so for two decades Schmeidler's conclusion about the meditation and psi relationship remained the best guess. Our more recent experiments involving meditators produced results consistent with the idea that meditation practice improves psi performance, but we haven't yet focused on explicitly testing different meditative techniques or exploring if the amount of meditation practice is correlated with psi performance.

The lack of attention toward meditation as a possible modulator of psi ability might be one of the reasons that the experimental outcomes we typically see in psi studies are much weaker than what is claimed in the yogic lore. Some of those differences may be due to embellishment of legendary stories about the siddhis, leading to inflated expectations about what is really possible. Another reason may be due to conducting psi studies with untrained people and in cultural contexts that are leery or frightened of psi phenomena.

What is needed to seriously study the meditation-siddhi-psi relationship is a systematic effort where we give the same psi tests repeatedly to experienced meditators in the same environments over an extended period of time. Those studies have begun.

Yogis and Tibetan Monks

In 2001, British psychologist Serena Roney-Dougal was invited to teach about psi research at Swami Satyananda Saraswati's Yoga University, called Bihar Yoga Bharati, in his ashram in Bihar, northeastern India. Roney-Dougal used that occasion to develop a research program with the yoga nuns and monks to study the relationship between meditation achievement and psi performance. Since then she and her colleagues have expanded their studies to include Tibetan Buddhists located at various monasteries in India.[169, 170, 339–341]

Similar to the yogic tradition, in Tibetan Buddhism it is understood that the siddhis arise only after one is able to sustain the deep absorption of samadhi. However, it is also recognized that not everyone who meditates will be able to achieve samadhi, nor will the siddhis that do arise necessarily be stable. As Roney-Dougal explained:

Tibetans separate two types of "clairvoyance." They consider that the one Western parapsychologists research is a low-level ability that is unreliable and subject to fraud. Many people are considered to have this ability and Tibetans consider that it is an inherent ability resulting from past life karma, which could, however, benefit from training by meditation.

The clairvoyance you attain after reaching Samadhi is a high level ability which is reliable. In interviews with various monks, it was stressed over and over again that only a few people attain Samadhi and clairvoyant abilities, and even then the clairvoyance is no more than 80% reliable. Omniscience arises only with full enlightenment. Not everyone who practices meditation will attain Samadhi, so not everyone who practices meditation will become psychic.[169] (p. 163)

While very-high-functioning psi may be rare, even among meditators, the question that interested Roney-Dougal was more modest: Do increased levels of meditation practice correlate with increased psi performance? This ought to be the case if yogic teachings are correct, because a key consequence of yogic practice is to bring to the surface skills that are inherent in everyone.

Roney-Dougal tested meditators with different levels of practice using the same psi test. To reduce environmental and procedural variations between sessions, she tested people at the same time of day, in the same location, and with the same timing between sessions (usually daily). She also presented the instructions for the experiment translated into the local language through an audio recording.

Roney-Dougal's standardized psi test was presented on a laptop computer. The meditator began each session with five minutes of relaxation followed by stating the intention to become aware of a photo that they would see on the laptop after a short meditation period. This was followed by fifteen minutes of meditation, and then the meditator was instructed to allow their mind to go blank and to allow target-related impressions to arise over the next four minutes.

After this they described their impressions and sketched whatever came to mind. Then they were shown four photos on a computer monitor. The pool of four images was randomly selected by the computer from a set of twenty-five groups of photos, where, as in the ganzfeld telepathy test, each group contained four photos that were as different from one another as possible.

Participants viewed the four photos together or separately on the laptop screen for as long as they wished. When ready to continue, they rated each photo on a hundred-point rating scale according to how confident they were that the image matched their earlier impression. At this point, if the trial was a precognition task, then after they entered their impression the computer would randomly select a target image and display it. If it was a clairvoyance task, then the computer displayed the target photo that it had selected at random when the session began. After each meditator completed eight sessions, he or she filled out a meditation attainment questionnaire.

Roney-Dougal used this test design because the Tibetan people have a long tradition of accepting precognition in the form of oracles and divination performed by the lamas (advanced monks). Clairvoyance is also culturally accepted as a key means for locating reincarnated monks (known as *tulkus*).

Over the course of six years, with the blessing of the Dalai Lama and Swami Satyananda, Roney-Dougal tested visitors, students, sanyasins (students who have taken some degree of yogic initiation), monks, nuns, rinpoches (believed to be reincarnated Tibetan lamas), lamas (advanced Tibetan monks who have completed a three-year retreat), and geshes (monks with the equivalent of a doctorate degree in Buddhist philosophy). She conducted two experiments in the yoga ashram and two more in various Tibetan monasteries, involving a total of fifty-two yogis and twenty-eight Tibetan monks.

The outcome of the experiments in the yoga ashram showed modest evidence that the longer the meditation practice, the better the psi scores, with odds against chance of 33 to 1. The tests at the Tibetan monasteries provided stronger results, with odds against chance of

2,000 to 1. When the data from both series of tests were combined, the odds against chance for the meditation-psi relationship were clearer, with odds against chance of 8,500 to 1. Combined with the earlier meditation-psi experiments, it appears that meditation does indeed lead to improved psi performance, and thus the *Yoga Sutras'* prescription for developing the siddhis is increasingly plausible.

Dalai Lama

Even given positive results of experiments, it is exceedingly difficult for the Western-acculturated mind to accept that supernormal abilities really do exist. The Dalai Lama is often asked about this issue, and he wrote about it in his autobiography:

> Many westerners want to know whether the books on Tibet by people like Lobsang Rampa and some others, in which they speak about occult practices, are true. They also ask me whether Shambala (a legendary country referred to by certain scriptures and supposed to lie hidden among the northern wastes of Tibet) really exists. . . .
>
> In reply to the first two questions, I usually say that most of these books are works of imagination and that Shambala exists, yes, but not in a conventional sense. At the same time, it would be wrong to deny that some Tantric practices do genuinely give rise to mysterious phenomena.[6]

This statement is cautiously worded, and appropriate for a spiritual leader who was also a political leader for many years. The upshot of his answer is that yes, advanced meditative practices do give rise to some strange effects, and for the most part these practices have been ignored by science.

The Dalai Lama has been personally interested in promoting

science-spirit dialogues, but at the beginning these talks were not easy to arrange, even for him. Within meditative traditions advanced methods are considered a secret doctrine, and as we've seen repeated in the *Yoga Sutras*, demonstrating one's abilities for secular reasons is strongly taboo. Nevertheless, the Dalai Lama believed it was important to get science to investigate these phenomena:

> I hope one day to organise some sort of scientific enquiry into the phenomenon of oracles, which remain an important part of the Tibetan way of life. Before I speak about them in detail, however, I must stress that the purpose of oracles is not, as might be supposed, simply to foretell the future. This is only part of what they do. In addition, they can be called upon as protectors and in some cases they are used as healers. . . . Through mental training, we have developed techniques to do things which science cannot yet adequately explain. This, then, is the basis of the supposed "magic and mystery" of Tibetan Buddhism.[6] (p. 220)

Progress

A new wrinkle in the meditation-siddhi-psi relationship appeared in a meta-analysis of meditation studies, published in 2012 by Peter Sedlmeier of Chemnitz University of Technology (Germany) and his colleagues in *Psychological Bulletin*.[47]

Sedlmeier's meta-analysis sought to answer if meditation has positive effects. The outcome was a remarkably clear yes. Meditation has a "substantial impact on psychological variables" (p. 21). A second question asked if meditation is practically meaningful—that is, are the effects strong enough to provide therapeutic benefits? The answer again was a solid yes. The effects are comparable to standard behavioral and psychotherapeutic treatments. A third question asked if meditation was basically just a relaxation technique. The answer was that meditation is *not* just a relaxation technique, although there might be some commonalities in the two methods. So far, so good. This comprehensive meta-analysis rigorously confirmed what many meditation researchers had long suspected. Meditation works. But there was a new element in the discussion section of this article, a topic that is usually glossed over or completely missing from most academic studies of meditation: It addressed the siddhis, without apology.

This is more notable than it may seem. In our earlier chapters, we've seen many examples of scientific prejudice against the possibility of psi phenomena. That prejudice has led many scientists and scholars to avoid mentioning the siddhis.

But here is an article, published in a well-regarded mainstream psychology journal, mentioning the siddhis without immediately begging forgiveness. The siddhis are a core component of most meditative traditions, so one would think that any serious research on this topic would *have* to include a discussion of the siddhis. But most haven't, and the abyss is especially conspicuous in the neurosciences, where merely mentioning this topic in a positive tone is strictly forbidden.

Refreshingly, Sedlmeier writes:

In the introduction, we derived one general prediction for beginning and intermediate practitioners of meditation from both the Hindu and Buddhist approaches (meditation yields generally positive psychological effects), but we did not deal with predictions that refer to advanced or final stages in the meditation practice. Here is such a prediction. Both Hindu and Buddhist approaches hold that practitioners of meditation might develop a kind of supercognition, special abilities (*siddhis*) that exceed our normal abilities.

Buddhist theory predicts that six kinds of siddhis might arise. . . . Notably, the least spectacular one, destruction of the defiling impulses, is seen as the most significant. The others are psychokinesis, clairaudience, telepathic knowledge, retrocognitive knowledge . . . , and clairvoyance. The *Yoga Sutras* report more of these siddhis as a result of extended yoga practice. In both the Hindu and Buddhist approaches, siddhis are not regarded as very important, and the Buddha, as well as famous yogis, has warned of the dangers inherent in the siddhis. . . .

Nonetheless, a theory about the effects of meditation would not be complete without consideration of these altered states of consciousness. There is some evidence that such states can occur spontaneously . . . , but the effects found in meta-analyses are usually quite small. . . . To the best of our knowledge, nobody has yet examined whether the respective effects are more pronounced for experienced practitioners of meditation, as both the Hindu and Buddhist approaches would predict.[47] (p. 23)

As noted earlier in this chapter, Serena Roney-Dougal found that more advanced meditators did perform better on precognition tests, and in general the psi literature does indicate that meditators perform better. This supports Sedlmeier's prediction about the effects of advanced stages of meditation practice, and once again we find that Patanjali is correct.

Summary

So far, we've learned that there are rational, evidence-based reasons to accept that some of the siddhis—the ones that have been repeatedly tested under controlled conditions—are real. We've seen evidence suggesting that advanced meditation may be associated with improved psi performance. And, except for rare individuals and some advanced meditators, among the general population we've seen that these abilities tend to be weak, sporadic, and uncontrollable.

From a scientific perspective, the mere *existence* of these phenomena, regardless of how weak or unreliable they may be, is astounding. It tells us that the modern understanding of the human mind, which is based on the neurosciences and its approach to studying brain function, has completely overlooked a fundamental aspect of our capacities and potentials. It says that both science and religious scholarship have prematurely discarded stories about the siddhis as mere superstitions. Undoubtedly many of those legendary tales are pure fantasy. But we now know that *some* of them described dazzling gems that have been obscured by the distortions of history. Identifying and polishing those gems with modern techniques opens the real possibility of discovering whole new realms of knowledge.

Over time, as mainstream interest in studying the capacities of advanced meditators increases, we are likely to understand psi and the siddhis in new ways. As that happens, more integrated models of reality will arise, and eventually technologies may be developed. How long do we have to wait before this knowledge is pragmatically useful? Not too long.

PART III

. . . And Beyond

After gaining confidence that some of the yoga superpowers are real, what does this tell us about the scintillating boundary between the inner and outer worlds?

Science hasn't progressed very far into those rarified domains, so to extend our investigation we must now rely on possibilities and speculations beyond science and the siddhis.

CHAPTER 15

Pragmatics

Pragmatism asks its usual question: "Grant an idea or belief to be true," it says, "what concrete difference will its being true make in anyone's actual life? How will the truth be realized? What experiences will be different from those which would obtain if the belief were false? What, in short, is the truth's cash-value in experiential terms?"

—*William James*

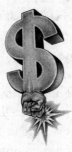

Tales of superpowers are one thing. Making money is another.

For those with no interest in cerebral issues like the ontological basis of reality, or spiritual issues like the path to liberation, there is one sure way to grab attention: Beat Wall Street.

Siddhis on Wall Street

Professional athletes have above-average physical capacities, but there's one key factor that discriminates between the competitor and the world champion: superior mental discipline. For years golfer Tiger Woods was the poster child for mental toughness. It is credited for his remarkable record of winning seventy-six Professional Golfers Association (PGA) tournaments as of spring 2013.

But after an infidelity scandal came to light in December 2009, Woods's mental edge was shattered and he soon dropped from the number one player in the world to fifty-eighth. Maintaining the extreme mental absorption necessary to win at the professional level in any sport is suggestive of the dedication and talent it takes to achieve samadhi. This raises the possibility that accomplished athletes might be good candidates for demonstrating psi.

Greg Kolodziejzyk is an Ironman triathlon competitor who holds world records on recumbent bicycles and pedal-powered boats, including the Guinness World Record for the greatest distance under human power in one day on land and water (647 miles on land, 152 miles on water). Unlike mere mortals, Greg is not fazed by major challenges, so he decided to see if he could use a precognitive form of remote viewing to outperform the futures market.[342]

He used a method known as *associative remote viewing*. Developed by anthropologist and explorer Stephan Schwartz,[343] this method is a way to optimize clairvoyance for use in practical applications. If the goal is to determine whether a certain stock will trade high or low, then trying to directly perceive the value of that stock with clairvoyance probably won't work.

Psychic information appears to be easier to gain in terms of perceptual primitives, such as shape, form, and color, rather than analytical factors such as precise location and specific words and numbers. This distinction is roughly similar to how the two hemispheres of the brain are specialized for different kinds of information processing.

In right-handed people, the left brain hemisphere is associated more with processing language and analytical and rational thinking, and the right brain hemisphere is associated more with form, symbolic, emotional, and intuitive thinking. In reality, the left brain–right brain distinction is an oversimplification of what is really going on, because in normal brains there is a huge amount of cross-talk between and within the hemispheres. But brain regions do process information differently, and because some of those differences appear to be related to perception of psi information, when it comes to using clairvoyance for practical purposes, it is necessary to use a trick.

The Trick

The trick works like this. First you ask an assistant to prepare many pairs of images, each image as different from the other as possible, and not to let you know what any of the images are so you won't be influenced by your preferences.

Say one pair of images consisted of a photo of an egg and a cactus. Now you have your assistant, or a computer program, randomly associate one image with a favorite stock going up in price on Friday, and the other image with the same stock going down in price on Friday. The association is used to eventually show you either a photo of an egg or a cactus depending on how the stock price moves on Friday.

Now imagine that it's Monday and you want to know how to prepare your stock trades before Friday. To do this you conduct a remote viewing trial where you imagine the image that you will be shown on Friday.

You meditate and empty your mind. After a while you gain a mental flash of something green and spiky. You record your impressions. Now you are shown two images. One is an egg and the other is a cactus. You assess how well your impression matches each image, and you decide with some confidence that you must have been seeing the cactus—it's green and spiky. Now you learn that the cactus image was randomly assigned to a drop in stock price, so you prepare your trade accordingly. Friday comes, the stock indeed drops, and you are shown the cactus image as feedback.

Making this type of trade based on a single remote viewing trial might work, but to increase the likelihood of making a correct decision you repeat this process many times and base your decision on the majority vote. You can also improve your decision by rating your confidence on each trial (before you see the target). If you perform several trials and you find that your remote viewing confidence is uniformly low, then you may decide to pass on that trade.

Starting in 1998, Greg Kolodziejzyk used an associative remote viewing technique to trade on the futures market. His computer-based method randomly picked from eight possibilities: S&P 500 index, US Treasury notes, wheat, oil, gold, Swiss franc, British pound, and the Canadian dollar. Then he selected a date in the future to enter and exit the trade. The range was from one day to two weeks in the future.

He conducted multiple remote viewing trials to develop a consensus decision to buy or sell, and the images he used for the remote viewing targets were selected from thousands of digital stock photographs from commercial sources, or were randomly selected images from the Internet.

To conduct a forecasting session, Greg took a few minutes to calm down, and then a few more to conduct the remote viewing task. He would conduct between five and ten remote viewing trials in a single session, so the whole process might take twenty or thirty minutes. In his words:

> My objective during this process is to generate random thoughts about the feedback image. I try to clear my mind, and think of nothing while imagining myself on the future feedback date and time, looking at a image on my computer screen. I sketch, or print any random thought that enters my mind. I ignore thoughts that seem like they were generated by my conscious mind and didn't seem random. I empha-

size thoughts that surprise me by how random they seem—especially if the thoughts are very detailed.

For example, recently during a remote viewing session, I thought of a small furry pet in my shirt pocket. This was a detailed perception, and seemed very random, so strong emphasis was placed on this perception in my resulting sketch. As it turned out, the feedback photo was a man holding a small dog over his shirt pocket.[344]

During the remote viewing process, Greg does not know what image is randomly assigned to the future buy (call this image A) or sell (image B) instruction. When he finishes all trials for a given trade, his computer automatically creates a combined score for image A and another score for image B, and the image with the highest score is the best prediction.

If the difference in scores between images A and B is large enough ("large enough" being determined based on his previous results), then he makes a trade. To prevent the decision to trade or not trade from being influenced by the behavior of the markets, he diligently avoids paying attention to the financial news in the days before the trade.

The Outcome

Using this method, over the thirteen years from May 1998 to September 2011, Greg made 285 trading attempts based on 5,677 associative remote viewing trials. Of those trials, 53 percent correctly predicted the behavior of the futures markets. Considered as a remote viewing experiment, this outcome is unlikely to occur by chance, with odds greater than 31,000 to 1. He also found that as his confidence in matching his impressions to the images improved, that his correct trading decisions also improved. At the highest level of confidence, his hit rate increased to 78 percent.

Among the 285 trading attempts, 181 led to decisions that provided confidence for Greg to feel comfortable enough to risk actual money. Those 181 trades were based upon 4,007 remote viewing trials, and 60 percent of the 181 trades were profitable. Starting with $50,000 in capital, his net profit was $146,000.

Other people have claimed to use associative remote viewing to beat the stock market.[329] Developed as a laboratory technique in the 1980s and known to just a few people at that time, some thirty years later a Google search on the terms "remote viewing" and "stock market" returns fifty-five thousand web pages; a more general search on the terms "remote viewing" and "applications" returns some seven hundred thousand web pages.

Very few of those pages report scientific studies, so all this should be taken with a grain of salt. It does, however, show widespread interest in what used to be a far-fringe esoteric topic. Among the few controlled studies that have been conducted, like Greg Kolodziejzyk's, the results confirm that people who are disciplined, persistent, and talented can make a profit in perceiving the future.

As to whether similar profits could have been made by having monkeys randomly toss darts at a list of stocks, in the case of the scientific tests we know exactly how unlikely this is. In Greg Kolodziejzyk's case, if we asked thirty-one thousand teams of monkeys to toss darts at stocks, and it was actually true that over the long term it is impossible for monkeys to outperform the stock market, then we would see results as good or better than Greg's just once.

And his profit speaks for itself.

Still, Greg Kolodziejzyk's case is not a fair test when it comes to the art of making money on Wall Street, because professional traders would never rely solely on psi to make a decision. They would make the best analytical choice they could based on the available information, and only then, faced with making a final decision without additional sources of information, they would turn to psi. That's where the extra factor might prove to be the difference between profit in the hundreds of thousands versus millions or more.

This same approach, using psi-mediated information when there are no other sources available, leads us to another viable application that addresses the "so what" question.

Psychic Detective

There are many accounts of psychic detective work and similar efforts by the US government's formerly secret psychic spy program.[327, 345, 346] From those cases it isn't possible to judge whether such skills are real or not because we're never told how many unsolved cases we're *not* hearing about. It's reasonable for a skeptic to assume that maybe now and then a psychic makes a lucky guess and helps to solve a case, and just as reasonable to assume that most of the time the guesses lead nowhere.

If that's all we knew about psychic abilities, it wouldn't give us much confidence about these stories. But given that we know from scientific experiments that clairvoyant abilities do exist, the assumption that psychic detectives and spies are *always* guessing is unjustified.

Beyond scientific reasons to accept that some cases of psychic detective work are valid, occasionally an example comes to light that is so remarkable that it deserves retelling. Such a case came to my attention as I was writing this chapter. It's an example of a psychic detective team that solved a crime that was rapidly headed toward the unsolved "cold case" files.

The crime concerns a con artist who was eventually convicted of murder. This case was reported in the *Las Vegas Sun* newspaper on May 5, 2012. The head of the remote viewing team that provided information that helped to crack this case is Angela Thompson Smith, a teacher of remote viewing and founder of the Nevada Remote Viewing Group.

I met Smith in the 1980s when she was on the staff at the Princeton (University) Engineering Anomalies Research Laboratory, and I was in the Psychology Department at the same university. Another personal connection to this case is Las Vegas–based photographer Robert Knight, whom I met in the late 1990s when he took my photo for a gallery he was creating, called the "Warrior's Path."

Knight became worried that he hadn't heard from a close friend of his for over a month, a well-known Denver radio personality named Stephen B. Williams. Knight knew of Angela Smith's interest in remote viewing, and so he asked her to help find his friend. Smith's team at the time consisted of six remote viewers besides herself. They included a retired airline captain, a retired US Air Force nurse, a civilian air force contractor, a civil engineer, a photographer, and a librarian.

Each person was assigned a random series of letters and numbers as the target. Unbeknownst to them this random "word" was linked to various aspects of the missing person case. Using a blinded target is an important element in remote viewing because it prevents the "viewers" (jargon for a remote viewer) from trying to guess the target. The viewers were asked to seek information about the missing man, about his location, and later about a profile of the murder suspect and where the suspect was located.

The composite information that they provided pointed to the missing man as dead, probably murdered on land and disposed of in the ocean, and possibly near Santa Barbara, California. Knight was understandably dismayed to receive this information, but he was even more upset when he learned from his wife that she had just seen a newscast about a decomposed, unidentified body found near Catalina Island, about twenty-two miles southwest of Los Angeles, and near Santa Barbara Island.

Based on the remote viewing information and his feeling of dread that it might be correct, Knight called the Los Angeles County morgue, which was holding the body. He told the skeptical clerk that the body might be missing three fingers from the left hand. (Knight's friend had lost three fingers in an accident in the ninth grade.) The clerk was shocked to find that the body was indeed missing those three fingers.

Further examination confirmed that it was Knight's friend; he had been shot in the head.

Knight instantly became a prime suspect in the murder, because how else could he have possibly known that this body was his friend? Fortunately, Knight knew a sheriff's department commander who was aware of the potential accuracy of remote viewing, and so he vouched for Knight, who was quickly cleared of suspicion.

Sergeant Ken Clark of the LA County Sheriff's Department later agreed that without Knight's information, and the scenario provided by the remote viewers, it would have been extremely difficult to identify the body because of its badly decomposed state.

With greater confidence, Knight then provided additional information supplied by Smith's team, including the suspect's identity. This was a man who was supposed to be investing his friend's money, but had actually stolen it. Unfortunately, the suspect was nowhere to be found. But again, Knight's information proved to be useful. Remote viewing suggested that the suspect had fled to the Caribbean islands. That turned out to be correct.

The suspect was then traced to Montana, where he was foolish enough to work for a boss who was a former cop. When the boss checked him out, he found that the suspect was wanted for questioning in this homicide. The suspect was ultimately arrested and convicted in 2011 and is now serving a life sentence.

Summary

What might Patanjali have said about using the siddhis to beat the stock market? I imagine he would have nodded and said yes, these abilities can be used to make money. But he might have added that for millennia advanced yoga techniques were kept secret because without substantial moral and ethical preparation most of us are just too immature to safely develop and use the superpowers. They'd end up being abused to inflate the selfish ego, or turned into weapons. And while solving crimes is an honorable profession, I suspect that Patanjali might have encouraged us instead to cultivate Sutra III.23: *Lovingkindness*, and to become a beacon of friendliness and goodwill to all. That would eventually preclude the need to solve crimes.

Beyond applications of the siddhis, what else do these abilities suggest?

CHAPTER 16

Future Human

Because politics is the art of the possible, it appeals only to second-rate minds. The first-raters . . . [are] only interested in the impossible.

—*Arthur C. Clarke,* The Fountain of Paradise

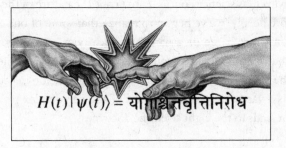

In this book we have explored a small portion of the scientific evidence associated with the supernormal abilities described in Patanjali's *Yoga Sutras.* Psi phenomena studied in hundreds of experiments by dozens of independent scientists over many years provide us with confidence that Patanjali wasn't spinning fairy tales.

For yogis and mystics this conclusion is obvious. For the dominant Western worldview it's a dilemma. As far as the scientific mainstream is concerned, if genuine siddhis exist, then some of the foundational beliefs underlying modern science are false. As we've seen, beliefs are exceptionally hardy, so it doesn't matter how much evidence is amassed in favor of the siddhis—scientific opinions will not change overnight.

But to see why science in the future will almost certainly accept some of the psi-oriented siddhis as self-evident, we need to better appreciate what's beneath today's resistance. To do this I'll briefly review what we might call the eightfold path of science. This involves eight doctrinal assumptions that underlie the present scientific view of reality.

The Eightfold Path

Assumptions in science don't just fall out of the sky. They are refined over centuries as a result of a great deal of experimentation, theoretical development, and hard thinking. So I'm not implying that the assumptions I'm about to recite are without justification.

However, as science continues to probe the nature of the universe ever more deeply, we've begun to realize that some of our earlier assumptions were based on a naive, "surface" view of reality. We now know that common sense—our everyday experience while driving down the street, talking to a friend, or buying a melon in the grocery store—is a vastly simplified snapshot of a hypercomplex reality. That snapshot leads to the eight scientific doctrines:

1. *Realism*: The physical world consists of objects that are completely independent of observation. This means, with a little exaggeration for the sake of illustration, that the moon is still there when you're not looking at it. This doctrine rules out the possibility that mind can directly influence matter.

2. *Localism*: Objects are completely separate. There is no such thing as "action at a distance." This excludes virtually all psi effects.

3. *Causality*: The arrow of time points exclusively from past to future, with no exceptions. This prohibits precognition.

4. *Mechanism*: Everything can be understood in the form of causal networks, like the gears of a clock that operate in a strictly local, causal

fashion. This does not abolish the possibility of psi phenomena, but it does limit viable theoretical explanations.

5. *Physicalism*: Everything can be described with real properties that exist in space and time, and all meaningful statements are either analytically provable, as in logic and mathematics, or can be reduced to experimentally verifiable facts. This does not necessarily limit the likelihood of psi effects.

6. *Materialism*: Everything, including mind, is made of matter or energy; anything else thought to be "immaterial" doesn't exist. It is not yet known that psi is necessarily immaterial, because the meaning of *material* has changed so much over the last century that it is not clear that this doctrine eliminates the possibility of psi phenomena.

7. *Determinism*: There is no free will, and all events are fully caused by preceding states. This doctrine casts doubt on the possibility of precognition and mind-matter interaction effects, but it doesn't prohibit them.

8. *Reductionism*: Objects are made up of a hierarchy of ever-smaller objects, with subatomic particles at the bottom. All causation is strictly "upward," from the microscopic to the macroscopic world. This allows matter-to-mind interactions, but excludes mind-to-matter interactions.

Most college students in the Western world are taught these doctrines throughout their formal education, but they are not often presented as assumptions. It is rare to find a student who recognizes that these ideas are guidelines and not self-evident facts of nature. As a result, students who become working scientists find no reason to question the assumptions. As physicist Anthony Leggett wrote, referring to just one of the doctrines, "It is difficult to exaggerate the degree to which reductionism is entrenched in the thinking not only of the twentieth-century physical scientist, but also to a large extent of the twentieth-century man in the street" (p. 4).[347] The same is still true for the twenty-first-century scientist, man, and woman in the street.

Unexamined assumptions in science can lead to problems when we're trying to understand the nature of reality and what is likely to be true or not true. Today we know that some of the resistance to psi and the siddhis has been based on false assumptions. That is, we know that *every single one* of the eightfold doctrines has been falsified by advancements in physics. For example, the doctrine of *realism* is falsified by quantum mechanics. That is, we know through theory and experiments that quantum objects do not have fully determined properties before they are observed.[348–350] *Causality* is falsified by general relativity, where a fixed arrow of time is known to be an illusion. *Locality* is falsified by quantum mechanics, in which quantum-entangled objects display "spooky action" at a distance and display instant correlations that are not located "inside" ordinary space-time.[351]

Physicalism, like realism, is falsified by quantum mechanics, partially because quantum events are not fully localized with real properties until they are observed, but more speculatively because of the possibility that "observation" *may* require consciousness, which in turn may or may not be a purely physical phenomenon. Experiments on mind-matter interaction, as discussed in earlier chapters, support this speculation.

Materialism, at least a simple physicalist form of materialism, looks like it may be headed for falsification if it turns out that psi phenomena cannot be accommodated by any known form of matter or energy. This is by no means certain yet, but the possibility remains. It may also fail because of quantum-inspired theories proposing that the physical world is better described in terms of mindlike *information* instead of material "stuff." For example, consider Princeton University physicist John Wheeler's famous concept of "it from bit":

Every "it"—every particle, every field of force, even the space-time continuum itself—derives its function, its meaning, its very existence entirely—even if in some contexts indirectly—from the apparatus-elicited answers to yes-or-no questions, binary choices, bits. "It from bit" symbolizes the idea that every item of the physical world has at bottom—a very deep bottom, in most instances—an immaterial source and explanation; that which we call reality arises in the last analysis from the posing of yes-no questions and the registering of equipment-evoked responses; in short, that all things physical are information-theoretic in origin and that this is a participatory universe.[352] (p. 5)

Or consider University of California psychologist Don Hoffman's more recent, radical theory of "conscious realism":

Despite substantial efforts by many researchers, we still have no scientific theory of how brain activity can create, or be, conscious experience. This is troubling, since we have a large body of correlations between brain activity and consciousness, correlations normally assumed to entail that brain activity creates conscious experience. Here I explore a solution to the mind-body problem that starts with the converse assumption: these correlations arise because consciousness creates brain activity, and indeed creates all objects and properties of the physical world. . . . *Conscious realism* states that the objective world consists of conscious agents and their experiences; these can be mathematically modeled and empirically explored in the normal scientific manner.[353] (p. 87)

Finally, *determinism* fails because of the collapse of causality, and *reductionism* breaks down because mind-body effects demonstrate "downward" causation from mind to body, and because psychokinesis demonstrates a more far-reaching form of downward causation, directly from mind to matter.

So now what? Scientific doctrines that were so successful in developing the modern worldview have turned out to be special cases of more comprehensive principles. The commonsense worldview has fallen apart.

One familiar reaction to radical change of any sort is panic. We see this panic expressed in the fierce denials printed on editorial pages, in journals, and in science magazines. A more optimistic approach is to look forward to radical changes (in ideas, anyway) with great excitement, because when fundamental worldviews change, *everything* eventually changes. What fun! New possibilities! New worlds to explore!

Quantum Inspirations

One possibility that suggests what the new worldview may look like is provided by recent discoveries and interpretations of quantum theory.[354] This discussion immediately gets us into dangerous territory, because foundational issues in quantum theory are still very much an open question, orthodox quantum theory does not allow for information transfer, and physicists don't like it when "quantum concepts" are, in their opinion, abused or misinterpreted. Nevertheless, we're in speculation mode, so let's see where it leads.

What may be poised to end the existence-of-psi debate is the growing acceptance of quantum biology. Articles on this topic can now be found in popular science magazines such as *Discover*, with feature stories like "Is Quantum Mechanics Controlling Your Thoughts?,"[355] and in *New Scientist*, with editorials such as "Quantum Biology Has Come in from the Cold."[356] The very idea that quantum theory would be relevant to biology was considered laughable nonsense just a few years ago. No one's laughing anymore.

The standard argument for why quantum mechanics and biology (especially the human brain) couldn't possibly have anything to do with each other is that quantum effects and biological activity are thought to occur at wildly different scales. Quantum theory is incredibly accurate in describing how objects behave at the nanometer scale (billions of a meter), in extremely cold conditions (near absolute zero), or at extremely fast rates (nanoseconds). By comparison biology is vastly bigger, hotter, and slower.

This distinction is important because the property of the quantum world associated with its spooky "nonlocal" character is called *coherence*. Maintaining quantum coherence is not easy to achieve in the laboratory because it is fragile and easily masked by interactions with the environment. So until recently, most physicists believed that quantum weirdness was acceptable in the microworld, but it had no bearing at all on the biological realm, and was thus completely irrelevant to the psychological domain.

These objections allowed neuroscientists to dismiss psi effects because it was assumed that the brain could be described flawlessly using plain old classical physics. And classical physics have no obvious mechanisms that could allow for the nonlocal connections that are the distinguishing feature of psi phenomena.

But those arguments were popular in the decade of the 2000s, which given today's scientific pace is already old news. A 2011 article in *Nature*, one of the top science journals, entitled "Physics of Life: The Dawn of Quantum Biology," explains why biology is not so separate from the quantum world after all:

> Discoveries in recent years suggest that nature knows a few tricks that physicists don't: coherent quantum processes may well be ubiquitous in the natural world. Known or suspected examples range from the ability of birds to navigate using Earth's magnetic field to the inner workings of photosynthesis—the process by which plants and bacteria turn sunlight, carbon dioxide and water into organic matter, and arguably the most important biochemical reaction on Earth.
>
> Biology has a knack for using what works, says Seth Lloyd, a physicist at the Massachusetts Institute of Technology in Cambridge. And if that means "quantum hanky-panky," he says,

"then quantum hanky-panky it is." Some researchers have even begun to talk of an emerging discipline called quantum biology, arguing that quantum effects are a vital, if rare, ingredient of the way nature works.[357] (pp. 272–73)

Also in 2011, physicist Vlatko Vedral of the Universities of Oxford and Singapore wrote in *Scientific American* that "quantum mechanics is not just about teeny particles. It applies to things of all sizes: birds, plants, maybe even people. . . . These effects are more pervasive than anyone ever suspected. They may operate in the cells of our body" (pp. 38–40).[358]

As some physicists had suspected, quantum effects do not magically disappear in larger systems. They are just more difficult to detect. But with newer techniques and measurement concepts, they are being found in increasingly larger and hotter systems.[359] This is leading to the expectation that there are deeper theories than quantum mechanics, and that when those are developed entirely new forms of postquantum spookiness will be found at all scales. As I described in a previous book, *Entangled Minds*, the direction that physics is headed is becoming increasingly compatible with the kind of physical reality that is required to support psi phenomena.

That is, common sense tells us that the everyday world is fixed in space and time. Our watches remind us of this, and we have to physically lug our bodies around to get from one place to the next. But within physics it is well established that beneath the appearances of common sense, space and time are *relationships* and not absolutes. We may be on the threshold of even more refined theories that redefine relationships as side effects arising out of a spaceless, timeless, informational reality.

If we didn't know better, we could imagine that this is what the yogis have been trying to tell us about the holistic nature of reality that they've experienced in samadhi. They just didn't have the technical language to describe it. As physicist Vedral says,

Space and time are two of the most fundamental classical concepts, but according to quantum mechanics they are secondary. The entanglements are primary. They interconnect quantum systems without reference to space and time.

If there were a dividing line between the quantum and the classical worlds, we could use the space and time of the classical world to provide a framework for describing quantum processes. But without such a dividing line—and, indeed, without a truly classical world—we lose this framework. We must explain space and time as somehow emerging from fundamentally spaceless and timeless physics.[358] (p. 43)

A half century ago, psi researchers were already proposing models based on quantum concepts.[1, 2, 295, 360, 361] It appears that the rest of the scientific world is beginning to catch up.

Toward a New Story

Millennia ago, everyday reality was regarded as a living, organic, conscious entity, permeated with minor and major deities who influenced all things. About five hundred years ago, with the rise of science, a new reality emerged and slowly transformed the old story into a mechanical, godless, mindless, isolated existence, crammed into a few dimensions of time and space.

That reality has been the dominant story for many generations now, and some aspects of it have proven to be fabulously productive. But at a cost. An increasingly troubling argument can be made that our existing worldview is also blithely leading humanity toward extinction as we move full speed ahead into a "tipping point" in the global ecosystem.[362, 363]

If civilization is fortunate enough to mature out of its infancy, then our scientific worldview will also have a chance to evolve into something new. That new story is not yet written, but visionaries are already beginning to describe reality in terms that echo key themes from more ancient times—reality as an interconnected, multidimensional, mindful, living, relational existence. And unlike the conceptual limitations faced by the earliest sages, this time we may be able to describe this reality using well-tested scientific ideas.[144, 364, 365] That is, maybe Patanjali laid it out thousands of years ago in 196 succinct sutras, but those aphorisms were written in a language that evolved during a prescientific era, so it did not contain many concepts about the physical world that are now reasonably well understood.

To gain a more comprehensive story of reality we need to integrate the best and most enduring ideas from both ancient and modern worldviews. One way to work toward that goal is to consider a simplified version of the four primary models of mind-matter interaction that have developed over millennia.[366]

Philosophy	Problem	Miracle
Dualism	Interaction	Yes
Materialism	Emergence	Yes
Idealism	Emergence	Yes
Panpsychism	Binding	Sort of

Dualism is the idea that mind and matter are completely different domains of reality. Mind is subjective, nonphysical, ethereal consciousness-related stuff, and matter is objective, hard physical stuff. This insight was promoted by French philosopher René Descartes. It exists in a slightly different form as Sankhya philosophy, which is regarded by many Indian scholars as the philosophical basis of yoga.

In Sankhya there are two fundamental aspects of reality: *prakrti* and *purusa*. Prakrti is the evolving, changeable physical world familiar to science, whereas purusa is permanent, unchanging, pure consciousness-as-such. Unlike Descartes's version of dualism, Sankhya maintains a tripartite model: matter, mind, and pure consciousness. Both matter and mind are considered prakrti, or part of the physical world. This is similar to the models developed by the modern neurosciences—the mind is a brain-mediated information processing machine. But the mind also enjoys awareness and consciousness. Thus in Sankhya philosophy the mind is the missing link between inanimate matter and conscious awareness. It is inseparably both at the same time.

Yoga seeks to purify that link so the relationship between the physical world and consciousness becomes clearer. In the process of clarification, the undistracted mind begins to see the true relationships between matter and consciousness, and as a side effect of that insight, the siddhis arise. When the link is completely clear, enlightenment is said to occur. That's the whole story of yoga in a nutshell.

The problem with both dualistic or tripartite philosophies is this: How can radically different domains interact at all? This is why philosopher Christian De Quincey calls dualism a miracle. At least within Sankhya the mind is regarded as consisting of both matter and consciousness, but that too doesn't cleanly solve the interaction problem.

The next major idea about mind and matter is *materialism*, which asserts that everything that exists, including mind and consciousness, consists of matter and energy. This is the dominant philosophy of science today, and it asserts that there is nothing special about consciousness because it is simply due to activity in the brain. The problem with materialism is that no one has any (good) idea how the mindless physical brain can give rise to subjective experience. This impasse has led some philosophers to sidestep the problem by simply denying that subjective experience exists. Within that rather odd view, we're all just zombies.[366-368]

The miracle of materialism is that somehow, magically, an insentient universe evolved into sentient beings. One explanation for this is that consciousness emerges as a result of the complexity and self-reflective recursion that is built into the circuits of the brain, like a hall of mirrors. But a hall of mirrors is not aware of itself (at least I hope not given the bleary eyes and ratty hairdos presented to innumerable bathroom mirrors in the morning), so the analogy is unsatisfactory.

Idealism is materialism upside down. It proposes that all that exists is pure consciousness. Everything in the physical world, all matter and energy, are emergent properties of consciousness. In its more radical form, it asserts that the entire physical world is a mind-generated illusion, somewhat like the virtual world in the movie *The Matrix*. Idealism runs into a miracle if it proposes that out of ephemeral nonphysical consciousness there emerges a hard, physical world. How does that happen? Once emerged, is it still connected to mind or does it go on its merry way? On the other hand, if it proposes that everything is an imaginary projection of consciousness, then the miracle is that everyone other than me is also a part of my imagination. Does that mean I still have to pay taxes?

Panpsychism is the fourth main worldview. It acknowledges that mind and matter are quite real, but it also proposes that these elements of reality are inseparable and go all the way down to elementary particles and "below," and also all the way up to the universe and beyond. The idea of a complementary relationship, where something is "both/and" rather than "either/or," is a core concept within quantum theory. Light, for example, behaves *both* as a wave and as a particle, depending on how you look at it. The advantage of panpsychism is that no miracles are required to account for how matter can be sentient, or how mind can have physical consequences. It is *both/and*.

But all is not completely rosy. The trouble with panpsychism is called the binding problem. This means that if all matter is already sentient, then every atom of your body, your cells, and your organs should also be sentient. Why then is your sense of self a unity and not a multitude? What binds it all together so that the "I" within you experiences just one self rather than trillions of tiny selves?

Dealing with the New Story

One of the more interesting takes on the developing new story of reality has been proposed by Rice University's Jeffrey Kripal, who, as a scholar of comparative religion, has explored the core themes of his discipline—the sacred, the paranormal, the supernormal, the mystical, and the spiritual—in a direction that few academics have dared to tred.[80] He views the intense popular interest in the paranormal as more than a mere fascination with fictional miracles, but rather as a sign of the original meaning of *fascination*—a bewitching accompanied simultaneously by awe and terror. He defines "psychic phenomena" as "the sacred in transit from a traditional religious register into a modern scientific one," and the *sacred* as

> what the German theologian and historian of religions Rudolf
> Otto meant, that is, a particular structure of human conscious-
> ness that corresponds to a palpable presence, energy, or power
> encountered in the environment. Otto captured this sacred
> sixth sense, at once subject and object, in a famous Latin sound
> bite: the sacred is the *mysterium tremendum et fascinans*, that is,
> the mystical (*mysterium*) as both fucking scary (*tremendum*) and
> utterly fascinating (*fascinans*). [80] (p. 9)

With the sacred viewed within this gripping, emotionally charged sense, it is hardly surprising that these topics are too disturbing to be studied either by religious scholarship or by science. The presence of real siddhis, real psychic effects lurking in the dark boundaries between mind and matter, are so frightening and disorienting that defense mechanisms immediately snap into place to protect our psyches from these disturbing thoughts. We become blind to personal psychic episodes and to the supportive scientific evidence, we conveniently forget mind-shattering synchronicities, and if the intensity of the *mysterium tremendum* becomes too hot, we angrily deny any interest in the topic while backing away and vigorously making the sign of the cross.

Within science this sort of behavior is understandable; science doesn't like what it can't explain because it makes scientists feel stupid. But the same resistance is also endemic in comparative religion scholarship, which is *supposed* to be the discipline that studies the sacred. As Kripal says, scholars of religion "simply ignore . . . or brush their data aside as 'primitive,' 'mistaken,' and so on. Now the dismissing word in vogue is 'anecdotal' " (pp. 17–18).[80]

One reason for this odd state of affairs is that real psi and real siddhis powerfully refute Descartes's dualism, the very idea that led to the split between science, which deals with matter, and the humanities, which deal with mind. This distinction has carved up the world so successfully that when phenomena appear that harshly illuminate the artificial nature of the split, the resulting glare, says Kripal, "can only violate and offend our present order of knowledge and possibility" (p. 24).[80]

From this analysis, Kripal arrives at his central argument: Psychic phenomena may be thought of as *symbols* that indicate "the irruption [a bursting in] of meaning in the physical world via the radical collapse of the subject-object structure itself. They are not simply physical events. They are also *meaning events*" (p. 25).[80] In other words, where objective and subjective meet, the fabric of reality itself blurs. This is a place that is not quite physical, and not quite mental, but a limbo that somehow contains and creates both. This sounds like a science fiction scenario gone mad, but according to Kripal:

> The new sensibility does not threaten a regression from rationality to superstition; rather, it allows for expansion beyond the one-sided worldview that scientism has provided us over the last three hundred years. We should never forget how utterly unsophisticated the tenets of eighteenth-century rationalism have left us, believers and unbelievers alike, in that complex arena we blithely dub "spiritual." . . . What our perspective does not allow us to recognize is the positive and enduring dimension of such ideas when they are consciously articulated

in our culture. We forget that Western culture is equally about Platonism and Aristotelianism, idealism and empiricism, *gnosis* and *episteme,* and that for most of this culture's history one or the other has been conspicuously dominant—and dedicated to stamping the other out.[80] (p. 59)

Consciousness as Glue

Max Planck, the originator of quantum theory, once said in an interview, "I regard consciousness as fundamental. I regard matter as derivative from consciousness. We cannot get behind consciousness. Everything that we talk about, everything that we regard as existing, postulates consciousness."[369] And Wolfgang Pauli, considered a towering genius by the other developers of quantum theory, noted: "It is my personal opinion that in the science of the future reality will neither be 'psychic' nor 'physical' but somehow both and somehow neither."[370]

A more recent contributor to this line of thinking is Stanford University physicist Andrei Linde, originator of the inflationary theory of cosmology, a leading contender for explaining how the Big Bang evolved into the universe that we observe today.[20] Linde points out, as have many others, that while physics is the study of the objective universe, it is known only through the subjective, our consciousness. This is so obvious that it is easily overlooked, and the omission leads many to the belief that consciousness is just another aspect of the inanimate matter that constitutes the rest of the universe. This deifies objectivity and it becomes difficult to imagine how things could be otherwise.

But it may be a mistake in the same sense that previous generations of physicists once thought that space and time were absolutes, or that matter and energy were obviously different. Linde speculates:

Is it possible that consciousness, like space-time, has its own intrinsic degrees of freedom, and that neglecting these will lead to a description of the universe that is fundamentally incomplete? What if our perceptions are as real [as] (or maybe, in a certain sense, are even more real) than material objects?[371]

In discussing this possibility, Buddhist scholar and physicist Alan Wallace points out that gravitational waves interact with matter so weakly that persuasive evidence that they even exist has yet to be found. But their existence is essential to uphold prevailing physical models of the fundamental particles. Wallace speculates: "Perhaps consciousness plays an equally important role in nature, despite the fact that it has been ignored until now in understanding well-studied physical processes in the brain and elsewhere" (p. 31).[20]

That is, could consciousness be a fundamental force in the universe that binds and shapes how the universe manifests? Like gravity, in the small scale it's too weak to be noticed, it simmers in the "background," it's too alien to our ordinary way of viewing the objective world to be able to detect. But it might be the glue that holds everything together and creates something rather than nothing.

A Symbolic Reality

Nobel laureate physicist Eugene Wigner marveled over the astonishing ability of mathematics—the symbolic language of science—to accurately describe the behavior of the physical world.[372] He noted that in spite of the baffling complexities of the world, some aspects are sufficiently stable that we've been lucky enough to identify "laws of nature." Without those regularities science would never have developed. Wigner believed it was not at all obvious or natural that such laws of nature *should* exist, much less that we've been able to discover some of them.

Like Wigner, mathematician Roger Penrose noted that some of the basic physical laws "are precise to an extraordinary degree, far beyond the precision of our direct sense experiences or of the combined calculational powers of all conscious individuals within the ken of mankind."[373] Penrose mentioned as an example Newton's gravitational theory as applied to the movements of the solar system, which is precise to one part in ten million. Einstein's theory of relativity improved upon Newton by another factor of ten million, and it also predicted bizarre new effects such as black holes and gravitational lenses. When astrophysicists went looking for these unexpected phenomena, to everyone's astonishment they found them.

Penrose then suggested that the amazing accuracy of the mathematical predictions "was not the result of a new theory being introduced only to make sense of vast amounts of new data. Rather, the extra precision was seen only *after* each theory had been produced."[373] One way of interpreting this is that pure mathematics is in contact with the realm of Platonic ideas and forms. This implies the independent existence of a purely mental, symbolic, or imaginal reality.

For those who insist that mind is nothing more than brain, mathematics is nothing more than the brain's representation of our observations of a preexisting physical world. But what happens when we unpack this argument? Mathematical symbols generated by three pounds of clockwork tissue somehow describe not only vast swatches of the physical universe to an inconceivable degree of precision, but they also predict phenomena that strongly contradict common sense, such as quantum entanglement and black holes. Those very same mathematical equations must necessarily include the behavior of the brains that created the mathematics in the first place.

How then is it possible for a lump of tissue to describe not only itself, but far more exotic realms with such stunning accuracy?

Could the universe be composed of a complementary substance that has both physical and mental aspects, similar to physicist David Bohm's idea of coexisting explicate and implicate orders? From this view, scientists seeking to confirm theoretical predictions based on pure mathematics will inevitably discover that the observable universe closely matches their predictions. Not because the mathematics are miraculous, but rather because expectations literally cause physical reality and its "laws" to manifest.

This outrageous idea borders on the New Age fantasy that if we only wished hard enough, then we could create our own reality. Hardly anyone takes this sort of radical solipsism seriously, except that it might just contain a kernel of truth. Perhaps some aspects of physical reality really are shaped by our expectations and intentions. Perhaps the fabric of reality is woven from the woof of matter/energy and the warp of mind. And when those threads are examined very closely, we find that they don't consist of ordinary stuff. They are made out of pure information.[374]

But instead of giving us grandiose superpowers promised by the ever-popular "law of attraction" or "power of positive thinking," we each have intentional *micropowers* that literally do shape the world we experience. Through future technologies, we may gain the ability to intensify these small effects, manifesting the promise of books like *The Secret* through something akin to the miraculous amplification technologies promoted by the lingerie chain Victoria's Secret.

Beyond such speculations, one thing is certain: Gaining a deeper understanding of consciousness will play an increasingly important role in twenty-first-century science. If the evolution of knowledge in this century exceeds that of the last, which seems likely, then we can look forward to a future that's likely to redefine our concepts of reality far beyond any of the strangest concepts we've encountered so far.[375]

Where Inner and Outer Space Meet

Reality built out of imagination, which in turn is a manifestation of a primordial "substance" that is both mind and matter? It sounds like science fiction. But there is evidence that this may be so, and if true, it might explain a number of persistent puzzles, from legends of the siddhis, to psi in life and the laboratory, and even, as unlikely as it may seem, to "unidentified flying objects" (UFOs).

Historical analyses of UFO cases, such as those recited in Richard Dolan's comprehensive books, *UFOs and the National Security State*[376] and *The Cover-Up Exposed*,[377] leave little doubt that something peculiar has been going on in the skies (and occasionally in the oceans) for many years, and that no one seems to have a clear idea about what *it* is. Some of the unexplained cases may be due to secret tests of aircraft or spacecraft, but that doesn't fully explain the mystery because objects displaying outrageous flying maneuvers were reported long before we (humans, at least) had aircraft.[378]

Whatever is happening, the discomfort is heightened when we consider the UFO's enigmatic cousins: crop circles, animal mutilations, men in black, purported alien abductions, and so on. Some reports of these phenomena are undoubtedly hoaxes. But all of them? The same has been claimed about psi phenomena, and scientific tests now tell us that such facile dismissals are invalid. It leads us to the conclusion that *some of these enigmas might be real.*

Here's where the phenomenological complex begins to bear a resemblance to otherworldly experiences reported in yogic, shamanic, psychedelic, mystical, and psychic states, and to folklore, mythology, and religious lore. Could these apparently disparate phenomena, many of which have been tossed into the "paranormal" wastebasket, be connected in some way?

Rise of the Imaginal

The modern era of the "flying saucer" began in June 1947 when pilot Kenneth Arnold saw a series of flying disks performing strange maneuvers, "like," he said, "a saucer would if you skipped it across the water." The June 26, 1947, issue of the *Chicago Daily Tribune* quoted Arnold. He added, "I saw . . . a series of objects that were traveling incredibly fast. They were silvery and shiny and seemed to be shaped like a pie plate."

Thirty years before Arnold's miracle, a similar sky-based miracle was reported in Fatima, Portugal. Three children reported that they were being visited by the Blessed Virgin Mary. In September 1917, thousands of witnesses reported seeing something arrive in an "aeroplane of light," an "immense globe, flying westwards, at moderate speed."[77, 378] The following month, the crowd had swelled to seventy thousand witnesses. One of them, a Professor Almeida Garrett of Coimbra University, later wrote:

> Suddenly, the sun shone through the dense cloud which covered it: everybody looked in its direction. It looked like a disc, of a very definite contour. . . . This clear-shaped disc suddenly began turning. It rotated with increasing speed. Suddenly, the crowd began crying with anguish. The sun, revolving all the time, began falling towards the earth, reddish and bloody, threatening to crush everybody under its fiery weight.[77]

Such experiences are not reported as fantasies, but they do seem to be interpreted in accordance with the observer's expectations. Religious pilgrims at Fatima interpreted a disk in the sky as a religious miracle; Kenneth Arnold saw flying aircraft; people in the US Midwest in the late nineteenth century saw flying schooners.[379, 380] Others may perceive ghosts of the dead, apparitions of the living, fairies, or "orbs" of intelligent light. Westerners today tend to see technologically sophisticated spacecraft piloted by humanoids, straight out of central casting for a science fiction movie. We expect to get radar hits on solid flying machines, and sometimes we do.

One of the first to explore the theme of mythology manifesting as real was psychoanalyst Carl Jung, who in 1957 published the book *Flying Saucers: A Modern Myth of Things Seen in the Sky.*[381] More recently, computer scientist Jacques Vallee,[378] author Keith Thompson,[382] and folklorists Peter Rojcewicz and Thomas Bullard[383] have written about the parallels among UFOs, folklore, and mythology.

Jung's use of the term "myth" does not imply that UFOs sightings, or for that matter encounters with angels, aliens, fairies, sprites, elves, or demons, are just fantasies. Rather, it suggests that some of these experiences may literally be psychophysical, a blurring of conventional boundaries between objective and subjective realities.

Some may object that this proposal doesn't account for the physical traces associated with some UFO reports. But that misinterprets what Jung and others have proposed. They suggest that the manifest world emerges from mind. That is, that *mind literally shapes matter*, that the imaginal and the real are not as separate as they seem. Where have we heard that before?

Mind Change

Former president of the Institute of Noetic Sciences Willis Harman discussed three basic ways of looking at the world in his book *Global Mind Change*.[384] He called the current Western scientific worldview *materialistic monism*. Within this worldview, everything is made out of a single substance: matter (and energy). From matter emerges everything, including the brain-generated illusion called mind.

For those who are firmly entrenched within the grasp of materialistic monism, angels and aliens walking through walls are acceptable plots for a fantasy story, but they are impossible in the real world. Likewise, real UFOs are conceivable, but only in terms of hard, physical spacecraft with humanoid pilots. Most of modern technology was created based on materialistic monism, so it carries enormous persuasive power. But those annoying anomalies keep popping up, from the yogic siddhis to the panoply of psi experiences, suggesting that this worldview is incomplete.

Harman's second worldview was *dualism,* which assumes two fundamentally different kinds of substances in the universe: matter and mind. As noted earlier, most scientists today reject dualism because it begs the problem of how two completely different substances could ever interact. This problem may be partially overcome from the Sankhya philosophy perspective, where mind is a complementary entity with both subjective and objective properties.

Harman's third worldview was *idealism,* or mental monism, which he argued was both the source of the perennial wisdom and the emerging worldview of the twenty-first century. From this perspective, consciousness is primary, and matter and energy are emergent properties of mind. This worldview accommodates everything that materialistic monism and dualism allow, but it also accommodates rogue phenomena like the siddhis, observation-shy UFOs, and field consciousness effects.

If Willis Harman's intuition was correct, and as a species we are evolving toward a new fundamental worldview, then our interpretation of phenomena that lay in the boundaries between mind and matter may be headed toward a unification. If that does occur, then how that future world may look and feel stretches the imagination.

But perhaps this transformation is precisely what the mystics have been preparing us for so diligently. Maybe the experiences of samadhi and the siddhis are seen as ineffable and mysterious not just because we don't have the language to talk about them yet, but because if we really understood these concepts, *it would change everything.*

• • •

This is not the end of the story. In some ways, yogic knowledge is thousands of years ahead of where science is today. The development of refined introspection by generations of disciplined minds has presented solutions to problems about subjectivity and awareness that science continues to struggle with from the "outside." To gain a better foothold on the nature of consciousness, we may have to approach this issue more seriously from the "inside."

When science begins to consider the full range of phenomena associated with ancient contemplative practices, and when advanced practitioners of those methods begin to embrace the value of objective scientific studies, both traditions are likely to benefit. There are a few fledgling research programs aimed at achieving this integration, but the mainstream is mostly burdened with aged prejudices and the woo-woo taboo, and it's not quite ready to go there yet.

What might happen when this ancient-modern integration becomes a reality? On the beneficial side we can anticipate improved health care through a vastly better understanding of the mind-body relationship. We may see development of technologies that treat aspects of the mind-body system that are well understood in the wisdom traditions but are ignored by Western medicine (for the most part). This includes phenomena such as "subtle energies." We may see a substantial reduction in interpersonal conflict through a broader recognition of the interconnectedness of all life. As the boundaries between subjective and objective realities are better understood, the communications and energy industries may be radically altered.

On the other hand, we are likely to find that some aspects of the wisdom traditions are seriously distorted and in some cases are dangerously wrong. We may find growing societal resistance at the prospect of being "absorbed" into an increasingly powerful collective mind. And we may pass through a time when horrifically powerful weapons are created that reshape space-time and possibly even alter history.

As science and society begin to appreciate that some of the siddhis are real, and that other aspects of yogic lore also provide legitimate road maps of reality, we can anticipate that some scientists and scholars, especially those who have bet their careers on past theories, will become increasingly marginalized and resentful. But the teeth grinding will eventually settle down as younger investigators, who were not so entrenched in passé prejudices, reach their prime.

From what I've seen in recent years, this transition has already begun. When it reaches fruition, humanity may finally find itself at childhood's end.

I am grateful to many foundations and organizations for generously supporting my scientific research. They include the Federico and Elvia Faggin Foundation, the Fetzer Franklin Fund of the John E. Fetzer Memorial Trust, Fetzer Institute, Mental Insight Foundation, Interval Research Corporation, HESA Institute, Samueli Institute, Parapsychological Foundation, Bigelow Foundation, Richard Hodgson Memorial Fund of Harvard University, Bial Foundation (Portugal), Swedish Society for Psychical Research, Society for Psychical Research (England), Institut für Grenzgebiete der Psychologie und Psychohygiene (Germany), and the Indian Council for Philosophical Research. I'd also like to thank Richard and Connie Adams, and Claire Russell, for their support.

Over the years I've encountered a few managers and administrators whose sole interest was to maintain the status quo by avoiding controversy at all costs. Fortunately, I've met many more who understood the value and the risk of investigating beyond the known.

I thank my colleagues at the Institute of Noetic Sciences for creating a gracious and cooperative environment. For offering materials or comments on a draft of this book I wish to especially thank Michael Bloch, William Braud, Joseph Burnett, Arnaud Delorme, Michael Grosso, Robert Hogan, Greg Kolodziejzyk, Jeffrey Kripal, Andrea Livingston, Jenny Matthews, Leena Michel, Julia Mossbridge, Alan Pierce, Serena Roney-Dougal, Suman Sankar, Stephan Schwartz, Angela Thompson Smith, Patrizio Tressoldi, Jessica Utts, and Cassandra Vieten. I am also grateful for Selma Syrek's superb original illustrations, to my editor Gary Jansen, and to Deepak Chopra.

CLAIRVOYANCE: Ability to gain information from hidden or distant objects, without the use of the ordinary senses; unbound by the usual constraints of space and time.

ESP: Extrasensory perception, a traditional term for clairvoyance.

PARAPSYCHOLOGY: Twentieth-century term referring to the scientific study of psi phenomena.

PRECOGNITION: A form of clairvoyance when the object of perception is distant in time.

PSI: Letter "p" in the Greek alphabet, first letter in the word *psyche*, meaning mind or soul; refers to clairvoyance, precognition, telepathy, and psychokinesis; psi is not an acronym, it is not capitalized, pronounced "sigh."

PSYCHIC PHENOMENA: Popular term for psi phenomena.

PSYCHICAL PHENOMENA: Nineteenth-century term referring to the scientific study of psi phenomena.

PSYCHOKINESIS: Influence of mind on matter without the use of known forces. PK for short.

REMOTE VIEWING: Euphemism for clairvoyance, sometimes associated with a specific training process.

RNG: Random number generator, an electronic circuit designed to produce sequences of truly random bits (0s and 1s), based on a physical source of random events; used in the study of small-scale psychokinesis.

SAMADHI: Sanskrit term for a meditative state where ordinary distinctions dissolve into a deeply absorbed unity. Often described as an ecstatic or blissful state.

SAMYAMA: Sanskrit term for the combination of concentration, meditation, and samadhi, from which siddhis arise. This is occasionally spelled "sanyama."

SIDDHI: Sanskrit term for perfection or attainment, referring to legendary supernormal abilities said to be attainable through advanced meditation, repetition of mantras, drugs, or birth (i.e., natural talent).

SUPERNATURAL: Beyond the natural world; divine or godlike.

SUPERNORMAL: Aspects of nature that are not yet well understood; superior to normal, but not supernatural.

TELEPATHY: Mind-to-mind communication; not "mind reading."

xviii   **What is said to be unified** There are many interpretations of the experiences of *illumination* and *the Self*, with variations depending on factors such as context, culture, and religious framework.

xix   **A Harris poll in 2009** www.harrisinteractive.com/vault/ Harris_Poll_2009_12_15.pdf; accessed August 21, 2012.

xix   **A CBS News poll conducted** www.cbsnews.com/2100 -500160_162-507515.html; accessed August 21, 2012.

xxi   **I was invited by** I am grateful to Dr. K. Ramakrishna Rao, chairman of the council at the time, for nominating me for this honor.

4   **Given the glowing praise** For example, see the book *Train Your Mind, Change Your Brain*, by Sharon Begley, a science columnist for the *Wall Street Journal* and former senior science writer at *Newsweek*.

6   **Techniques used to achieve** There are many terms used to describe yoga powers. They include *jnana, aisvarya*, and *vibhuti* in the *Yoga Sutras*; *iddhi* and *rddhi* in Buddhist Sanskrit; *bala* in the *Mahabharata*; and *adhisthana* and *vikurvanain* in Mahayana Buddhism.

9   **In fact, most cultures** Gallup poll: "Three in Four Americans Believe in Paranormal"; http://www.gallup.com/poll/16915/ three-four-americans-believe-paranormal.aspx, accessed June 3, 2012.

9 **Many scientists and scholars** Ironically, the ancient Greek philosophers who developed the concept of superstition did so not to dismiss religious beliefs, but as a rhetorical weapon to ridicule those who insisted that the gods were capricious or immoral. The philosophers reasoned that the gods were superior beings and thus they obviously couldn't be influenced by menial sacrifices or other simple offerings. And thus the superstitious were those who believed that the gods displayed human weaknesses.

12 **If you look up** http://books.google.com/ngrams, accessed May 8, 2012.

15 **"100 Best Spiritual Books of the [20th] Century"** See http://www.gradresources.org/worldview_articles/book.shtml, accessed September 1, 2012.

17 **"Today we are dedicating"** See http://pentagonmeditationclub.com/history_about_us.htm, accessed August 24, 2012.

17 **In 1976, a Pentagon Meditation Club** See http://pentagonmeditationclub.com/history_timeline.htm, accessed August 24, 2012.

20 **Despite the good preachers' concerns** While yoga as a practice is not a conventional religious activity because it doesn't rely on faith, the goal of the yogic path is to achieve what could be commonly regarded as a religious experience. Some may report this experience as an impersonal Universal Self; others may encounter a personalized deity or God.

22 **The Institute of Noetic Sciences** See www.noetic.org and especially http://noetic.org/meditation/, accessed June 6, 2012.

24 **the Indian government has been busily codifying** See www.csir.res.in/External/Heads/TKDL/main_090209.HTM, or www.tkdl.res.in/tkdl/langdefault/common/Home.asp?GL=Eng, both accessed June 4, 2012. As of February

2009, the Indian Council of Scientific and Industrial Research has recorded 81,300 Ayurvedic formulations, 1,09,000 Unani (herbal) formulations, 12,200 compound formulations, and 500 yoga postures.

24　**She glamorized the practice** See www.nytimes .com/2002/04/30/world/indra-devi-102-dies-taught-yoga-to-stars-and-leaders.html, accessed June 4, 2012.

26　**But what we can't know** I am skipping over evidence for conscious experiences reported when the brain is no longer functioning. The growing literature on near-death experiences presents a major challenge to standard neuroscience assumptions about the relationship between brain and consciousness.

32　**the *odds against chance*** Odds against chance are more precisely expressed as $p/(1 - p)$ to 1, so in the case of $p = 0.05$ the odds would be 19 to 1. As p becomes smaller, this expression rapidly approaches the simpler and more intuitive $1/p$. I've found that for nonstatisticians odds are much easier to understand than p values.

32　**This is referred to** Academic jargon is oftentimes unnecessarily complicated. If I were writing a book about how to cure insomnia, I would use much more jargon.

36　**"Eighty-three hallucinating"** He was referring to the eighty-three disciples of Zen master Hakuin, and not to paranoid patients.

38　**This was literally a shift** In this sense the word *meta* refers to something that refers to itself, often at a higher level, thus meta-analysis is an analysis of analyses, meta-cognition is thinking about thought, meta-theory is a theory for specifying theories, meta-language is a language used to discuss language, etc. In this way metaphysics can be interpreted as the physics or the mathematical formalisms that are used to understand physics.

39   **The use of psychedelic drugs** This idea comes mainly from psychedelic researchers; many yogic scholars would strongly disagree about the revealed origins of the Vedas.

47   **Whether it's the face of Jesus** See, for example, http:// stuffthatlookslikejesus.com/, accessed June 3, 2012.

63   **As described by Montague Summers** Published in 1950, the book by Montague Summers was entitled *The Physical Phenomenon of Mysticism*. There is another book by the same title, with much content overlap, by Herbert Thurston, published in 1952.

63   **Another interpretation is proposed** Reductionism is sometimes called "nothing but-ism," e.g., psychology is nothing but brain activity, brain activity is nothing but mindless biochemistry, etc.

70   **"The semiotics of *Star Trek*"** These titles are fictional, but academic interest in the intersections among popular culture, science fiction and fantasy, and mythology is a fascinating and, I think, important topic.

84   **A prominent skeptic** These and other laudable achievements are listed on Wiseman's website: http://richardwiseman. wordpress.com/about-me/, accessed August 26, 2012.

84   **He later clarified** See http://subversivethinking.blogspot .com/2010/04/richard-wiseman-evidence-for-esp-meets.html, accessed August 26, 2012.

95   **Stone carvings depicting figures** Another interpretation of those carvings is that there weren't many chairs back then, so it's conceivable that those images simply reflect how people commonly sat in those days—cross-legged on the floor.

95   **A universal "Self"** Not all theologians would agree. In fact, scholars hardly ever agree on anything.

96   **As such, the wisdom** Scholars will debate this point. There are many variations and emphases in yoga practice and

philosophy; nevertheless, one may argue that there are more similarities than fundamental differences. While narratives—legendary stories—tend to easily evolve over time as language and culture changes, some practices, including chants from the Vedas, tend to be preserved closer to their original form.

97   **The four parts of** The number of sutras and even the number of books (*padas*) in the original *Yoga Sutras* is not known for sure.

100   **Patanjali describes a method** This is not to be confused with Ashtanga yoga, a popular yoga style developed by Sri K. Pattabhi Jois. See www.ashtanga.com for details.

104   **In thirty-four sutras** What I'm presenting is the "impersonalist" interpretation of liberation. There are other philosophies that regard *moksha* as liberation and communion with the universal Self while retaining one's personality.

113   **It would manifest in** Incorruption in this context means that the body does not decay. There are a surprising number of historical examples where this phenomenon has been claimed to occur.

116   **Even then, it took** I mean this in the sense that most of physics and virtually all of engineering is about pragmatic descriptions and models. When it comes down to explaining exactly what magnetism is—its essence, how and why it exists at all—answers can only be expressed in terms of mathematical models that are approximations of the real world. At truly fundamental levels most, perhaps all, of nature remains a profound mystery.

135   **The rule of thumb for assessing** More precisely, Rosenthal's rule of thumb is $5k + 10$, where k is the number of known studies.

138   **fraction of the observed variation** Variance as used here is a statistical term; it refers to a standard method of assessing how much a given measure varies around its average value.

139   **structure of the universe rests upon 4 percent** See http://www.space.com/11642-dark-matter-dark-energy-4-percent-universe-panek.html, accessed June 8, 2012.

139   **Similarly, the scientific framework** See http://www.sciencedaily.com/releases/2007/07/070712143308.htm, accessed June 8, 2012.

142   **SRI International** At one time SRI was affiliated with Stanford University, and the acronym SRI referred to Stanford (University) Research Institute. When it became independent from Stanford University, the named changed to SRI International.

146   **The difference between these** To avoid violating parametric assumptions, the statistical methods more commonly used in this type of test are randomized permutation techniques.

153   **So from an orthodox** The same is true in all presentiment experiments. I've just emphasized this design element here.

159   **But in the meditator group** All statistics were based on conservative nonparametric methods and adjusted for multiple comparisons.

163   **(a) analyses that were preplanned** That is, no "data-snooping" was allowed.

167   **unconscious exposure before** The technical term is called "priming."

172   **Wagenmakers set these odds** The actual figure was associated with 10^{-20}, or odds of 99,999,999,999,999,999,999 to 1.

173   **It turns out that** He used a Cauchy distribution.

174   **This means that if** The Bayes factor in the Bem, Utts, and Johnson paper was conservatively calculated for a two-sided alternative. The example that I present here, of how a Bayes factor ought to influence prior beliefs, assumes a one-sided alternative.

181   **Now ask Gail** This trick works for native English speakers. It might not work for speakers of other languages.

189   **Hard-nosed skeptics** See http://deanradin.blogspot .com/2009/09/skeptic-agrees-that-remote-viewing-is.html, accessed June 9, 2012.

194   **How is it possible that highly educated scientists** It is invalid to use a null outcome in an experiment as proof that something does not exist.

196   **Of the seven meta-analyses** The 20 to 1 odds against chance refers to a meta-analysis by Milton and Wiseman, which claimed a failure to replicate the ganzfeld telepathy effect based on a subset of studies they had selected. Investigation of their method of analysis found that they had underestimated the actual effect, which was actually modestly but significantly positive.

196   **The one and only meta-analysis** Hyman was concerned with what he saw as possible randomization flaws, and with assessments of study quality. When discrepancies arise in analyses of the same literature, it is useful to consider the opinions of other reviewers who have the technical skills to assess the disagreements. In this case, as I described on page 83 of my book *The Conscious Universe*, ten psychologists and statisticians were asked to evaluate Hyman's negative meta-analysis along with Charles Honorton's positive meta-analysis. Not one of the reviewers agreed with Hyman, and of the ten reviewers, two statisticians and two psychologists who were not previously associated with this debate explicitly agreed with Honorton. The bottom line: Neutral expert reviewers all agreed that the data supported evidence for telepathy.

197   **Tressoldi found that** The analysis was conservative in the sense that it assumed that the effect size varied randomly across the studies.

199   **A series of clever experiments** See http://www.sheldrake.org /Articles&Papers/papers/telepathy/index.html, accessed June 9, 2012.

206   **"The only thing that"** See www.mentalhelp.net/poc/view_ doc.php?type=doc&id=30709&w=9&cn=116, accessed June 5, 2012.

233   **Two of the electronic RNGs** See http://www.aw-el.com/, accessed June 9, 2012.

236   **Chance expectation is zero** Also see the website http:// noosphere.princeton.edu/ for the Global Consciousness Project's latest results, accessed June 4, 2012.

239   **And indeed, if you track** One would actually observe a diffraction pattern in a typical double-slit system, but the basic idea is the same.

242   **The double-slit experiment** See http://physics-animations .com/Physics/English/top10.htm for an animation of the double-slit experiment, accessed June 9, 2012.

258   **The peak near the value 1** In the figure the values on the x-axis are called "wave numbers." Each wave number corresponds to a frequency decomposed by the Fourier transform, with lower numbers associated with slower frequencies and higher number with higher frequencies.

258   **To some people, this instruction** See http://www.youtube .com/watch?v=DfPeprQ7oGc, accessed June 9, 2012.

270   **They later expanded** You can download "Occult Chemistry" for free from the Gutenberg Project at this website: http:// www.gutenberg.org/ebooks/16058, accessed June 10, 2012.

278   **The meditator began** In some early trials the target was a video clip.

288   **But after an infidelity scandal** As of June 4, 2012, Woods has rebounded to number four in the world.

293   **This case was reported** See http://www.lasvegassun.com /news/2012/may/05/seeing-dead-people-remote-viewers-nevada-help-solv/, accessed June 10, 2012.

293   **Another personal connection** See http://www .bibliotecapleyades.net/imagenes_sociopol/warriorspath/ warriorspath.htm, accessed June 10, 2012.

295   **The suspect was ultimately arrested** As of June 2012, Smith continues to provide remote viewing training and applications work through her company, Mindwise Consulting, in Boulder City, Nevada.

303   **And classical physics have no** Some physicists believe that revisions to the laws of thermodynamics may allow for retrocausation, which would provide an opening for precognition.

307   **That's the whole story of yoga in a nutshell** This is, of course, a highly simplified version of Sankhya philosophy.

319   **When it reaches fruition** Read Arthur C. Clarke's *Childhood's End* or Robert A. Heinlein's *Stranger in a Strange Land* for science fiction projections of what happens next.

1. Radin DI. *The Conscious Universe*. San Francisco: HarperOne; 1997.

2. Radin D. *Entangled Minds*. New York: Simon & Schuster; 2006.

3. Rao KR. Taxonomy of consciousness. In: Srinivasan N, Gupta AK, Pandey J, eds. *Advances in Cognitive Science*. Vol 1. Los Angeles: Sage; 2008:383-243.

4. Murphy M. *The Future of the Body: Explorations into the Further Evolution of Human Nature*. New York: Tarcher (Penguin); 1993.

5. Jacobsen KA. Yoga powers and religious traditions. In: Jacobsen KA, ed. *Yoga Powers: Extraordinary Capacities Attained Through Meditation and Concentration*. Leiden, The Netherlands: Koninklijke Brill; 2012.

6. Lama D. *Freedom in Exile: The Autobiography of the Dalai Lama*. San Francisco: HarperOne; 1990.

7. Gross PR, Levitt N, Lewis MW, eds. *The Flight from Science and Reason*. New York: New York Academy of Sciences; 1996. Annals of the New York Academy of Sciences; No. 775.

8. Clay A. *Feet of Clay: A Study of Gurus*. New York: Free Press Paperbacks; 1996.

9. Broad WJ. *The Science of Yoga*. New York: Simon & Schuster; 2012.

10. Criswell E. *How Yoga Works: An Introduction to Somatic Yoga*. Novato, CA: Freeperson Press; 1989.

11. McIntyre D, Sauter M, Stockdale C. Top 10 things Americans waste the most money on. 2011; http://www.topstockanalysts.com/index .php/2011/02/28/top-10-things-americans-waste-the-most-money-on/, accessed February 18, 2012.

12. World Health Organization. *Global Status Report on Alcohol and Health*. 20 Avenue Appia, 1211 Geneva 27, Switzerland: WHO Press, World Health Organization; 2011.

13. Distilled Spirits Council of the United States. *Economic Contributions of the Distilled Spirits Industry*; http://www.discus.org/economics/, accessed February 18, 2012.

14. Guilfoyle J. *Campaign for Tobacco-Free Kids*. September 16, 2011; http://www.tobaccofreekids.org/, accessed February 18, 2012.

15. Bharati SV. *Yoga Sutras of Patajali*. Vol II. Delhi: Motilal Banarsidass; 2001.

16. Desai YA. *Amrit Yoga and the Yoga Sutras*. Rhinebeck, NY: Red Elixir; 2010.

17. Satchidananda SS. *The Yoga Sutras of Patanjali*. 16th printing ed. Yogaville, VA: Integral Yoga Publications; 2011.

18. Simon D. *The Yoga Sutras of Patanjali As-It-Is: Introduction, Commentaries, and Translation*. 2011; http://www.rainbowbody.net/HeartMind/Yogasutra.htm., accessed May 18, 2011.

19. Shearer A. *Effortless Being: The Yoga Sutras of Pantanjali*. London: Wildwood House Limited; 1982.

20. Wallace BA. *Hidden Dimensions: The Unification of Physics and Consciousness*. New York: Columbia University Press; 2007.

21. Haraldsson E. Representative national surveys of psychic phenomena: Iceland, Great Britain, Sweden, USA and Gallup's multinational survey. *J Soc Psych Res*. 1985;53(801):145-158.

22. Martin DB. *Inventing Superstition: From the Hippocratics to the Christians*. Cambridge MA: Harvard University Press; 2004.

23. Michel J-B, Shen YK, Aiden AP, et al. Quantitative analysis of culture using millions of digitized books. *Science*. (Published online ahead of print: December 16, 2010.)

24. Bardach AL. What did J. D. Salinger, Leo Tolstoy, and Sarah Bernhardt have in common? *Wall Street Journal*. March 30, 2012; Life and Culture.

25. Macdonald KS. Yoga philosophy: Lectures delivered in New York, winter of 1895–6 by Swami Vivekananda on Raja-Yoga, or conquering the internal nature. *Am J Theol*. 1898;2(2):402-405.

26. Yogananda P. *Autobiography of a Yogi* (reprint of original 1946 edition). Nevada City, CA: Crystal Clarity Publishers; 2003.

27. Love R. *The Great Oom: The Improbable Birth of Yoga in America*. New York: Viking Adult; 2010.

28. Room HoRM. Meditation Room. 1955; http://artandhistory.house.gov/highlights.aspx?action=view&intID=524, accessed February 13, 2012.

29. Lapham LH. There once was a guru from Rishikesh. *The Saturday Evening Post*. May 4, 1968.

30. Meditation clubs flourish from capital to Pentagon for dissolving tension. *New York Times*. October 26, 1976.

31. Bradee R. Hopeful place in Pentagon: Peace meditation room. *The Milwaukee Sentinel*. 1988; Editorial page:5.

32. Bowman JH. Transcendental meditation: Skeptic tries it, comes away a believer. *Los Angeles Times*. June 13, 1973.

33. Drug overdose, not meditation, apparently killed yoga teacher. *Los Angeles Times*. July 2, 1975.

34. Cox H. *Turning East: The Promise and Peril of the New Orientalism*. New York: Simon and Schuster; 1977.

35. Bush M, ed. *Contemplation Nation: How Ancient Practices Are Changing the Way We Live*. Kalamazoo, MI: Fetzer Institute; 2011.

36. Yoga and the devil: Issue for Georgia town. *New York Times*. September 8, 1990.

37. Press A. Southern Baptist leader on yoga: Not Christianity. October 7, 2010; http://www.foxnews.com/us/2010/10/07/southern-baptist-leader-yoga-christianity/, accessed January 14, 2012.

38. Stein J, Bjerklie D, Park A, Biema DV. Just say Om. *Time*. August 4, 2003.

39. Onion T. One in five women training to be yoga instructors. October 19, 2005; http://www.theonion.com/articles/report-one-in-five-women-training-to-be-yoga-instr,5049/, accessed February 11, 2012.

40. Rochman B. Samurai mind training for modern American warriors. *Time*. September 6, 2009.

41. Mead R. Maharishi prep. *The New Yorker*. March 22, 2004.

42. Cullen LT. How to get smarter, one breath at a time. *Time*. January 10, 2006.

43. Cloud J. Losing focus? Studies say meditation may help. *Time*. August 6, 2010.

44. Park A. Study: Yoga improves quality of life after cancer. *Time*. May 19, 2010.

45. Oz M. Medical meditation: Say om before surgery. *Time*. January 20, 2003.

46. Schwartz SA. Meditation—The controlled psychophysical self-regulation process that works. *Explore*. 2011;7(6):348-353.

47. Sedlmeier P, Eberth J, Schwarz M, et al. The psychological effects of meditation: A meta-analysis. *Psychol Bull*. May 14, 2012.

48. Ellison K. Giving meditation a spin. *The Washington Post*, January 23, 2007.

49. Singleton M. *Yoga Body: The Origins of Modern Posture Practice*. Kindle ed. Oxford, UK: Oxford University Press; 2010.

50. Devi I. *Forever Young, Forever Healthy*. Englewood Cliffs, NJ: Prentice-Hall; 1953.

51. Goldberg P. *American Veda: From Emerson and the Beatles to Yoga and Meditation; How Indian Spirituality Changed the West*. Harmony; 2010.

52. Public Education and Communication Committee. "Neuroscience Core Concepts." In: Society for Neuroscience, ed. *Neuroscience Quarterly*. 2007.

53. Chalmers DJ. *The Conscious Mind: In Search of a Fundamental Theory*. New York: Oxford University Press; 1996.

54. Beauregard M. *Brain Wars: The Scientific Battle over the Existence of the Mind and the Proof That Will Change the Way We Live Our Lives*. San Francisco: HarperOne; 2012.

55. Trimble MR. *Soul in the Brain: The Cerebral Basis of Language, Art, and Belief*. Baltimore, MD: Johns Hopkins University Press; 2007.

56. Urgesi C, Aglioti SM, Skrap M, Fabbro F. The spiritual brain: Selective cortical lesions modulate human self-transcendence. *Neuron*. 2010;65(3):309-319.

57. Ornstein R, Dewan T. *MindReal: How the Mind Creates Its Own Virtual Reality*. Boston: Malor Books; 2008.

58. Begley S. *Train Your Mind, Change Your Brain: How a New Science Reveals Our Extraordinary Potential to Transform Ourselves*. New York: Random House; 2008.

59. Kozhevnikov M, Louchakova O, Josipovic Z, Motes MA. The enhancement of visuospatial processing efficiency through Buddhist deity meditation. *Psychol Sci*. 2009;20:645.

60. Feuerstein G. *Yoga: The Technology of Ecstasy*. Los Angeles: Jeremy P. Tarcher; 1989.

61. Akiskal HS, Akiskal KK. In search of Aristotle: temperament, human nature, melancholia, creativity and eminence. *J Affect Disord*. June 2007;100(1-3):1-6.

62. Doerr-Zegers O. Phenomenology of genius and psychopathology. *Seishin Shinkeigaku Zasshi*. 2003;105(3):277-286.

63. Strassman R, Wojtowicz S, Luna LE, Frecska E. *Inner Paths to Outer Space: Journeys to Alien Worlds Through Psychedelics and Other Spiritual Technologies*. Rochester, VT: Park Street Press; 2008.

64. Walsh R. *The World of Shamanism: New Views of an Ancient Tradition*. Woodbury, MN: Llewellyn Publications; 2007.

65. Schrödinger E. *My View of the World*. Cambridge, UK: Cambridge University Press; 1964.

66. Wilber K, Stein FM. Quantum questions: Mystical writings of the world's great physicists. *Am J Phys*. 1985;53(6):601.

67. Barre WL. Shamanic origins of religion and medicine. *J Psychedelic Drugs*. 1979;11(1-2).

68. Feeney K. Revisiting Wasson's soma: Exploring the effects of preparation on the chemistry of Amanita muscaria. *J Psychoactive Drugs*. December 2010;42(4):499-506.

69. Harner MJ. *Hallucinogens and Shamanism*. London: Oxford University Press; 1973.

70. Herndon CN, Uiterloo M, Uremaru A, Plotkin MJ, Emanuels-Smith G, Jitan J. Disease concepts and treatment by tribal healers of an Amazonian forest culture. *J Ethnobiol Ethnomed*. 2009;5:27.

71. Pinchbeck D. *Breaking Open the Head: A Psychedelic Journey into the Heart of Contemporary Shamanism*. New York: Three Rivers Press; 2002.

72. Griffiths RR, Richards WA, Johnson MW, McCann UD, Jesse R. Mystical-type experiences occasioned by psilocybin mediate the attribution of personal meaning and spiritual significance 14 months later. *J Psychopharmacol*. 2008;22(6):621-632.

73. Coffey M. *Explorers of the Infinite*. New York: Jeremy P. Tarcher/Penguin; 2008.

74. Clark WH. Parapsychology and religion. In: Wolman BB, ed. *Handbook of Parapsychology*. New York: Van Nostrand Reinhold; 1977:769-799.

75. Inayat-Khan Z. Islamic and Islamicate contemplative practice in the United States. In: Bush M, ed. *Contemplation Nation*. Kalamazoo, MI: Fetzer Institute; 2011:97-98.

76. Forum P. Pew Forum on Religion and Public Life. 2007; Pew Forum. Available at http://www.pewforum.org/Age/Religion-Among-the-Millennials.aspx, accessed February 18, 2012.

77. Vallee J. *UFO's in Space: Anatomy of a Phenomenon*. New York: Ballantine Books; 1965.

78. Presence R. Real Presence Eucharistic Education and Adoration Association. 2012; http://www.therealpresence.org/eucharst/mir/a3.html, accessed April 4, 2012.

79. Weddle D. *Miracles: Wonder and Meaning in World Religions*. New York: NYU Press; 2010.

80. Kripal JJ. *Authors of the Impossible: The Paranormal and the Sacred*. Chicago: University of Chicago Press; 2010.

81. Einstein A. *The World as I See It*. New York: Philosophical Library; 1949.

82. Anatrella FT. The world of youth today: who are they and what do they seek? 2003; http://www.vatican.va/roman_curia/pontifical_councils/laity/Colonia2005/rc_pc_laity_doc_20030805_p-anatrella-gmg_en.html, accessed February 12, 2012.

83. James W. *The Varieties of Religious Experience.* New York: Random House; 1929.

84. Shook JR. *God Debates: A 21st Century Guide for Atheists and Believers (and Everyone in Between).* Hoboken, NJ: Wiley; 2010.

85. Studstill R. *The Unity of Mystical Traditions: The Transformation of Consciousness in Tibetan and German Mysticism.* Boston: Brill; 2005.

86. Lopez, DS Jr. *Buddhism & Science: A Guide for the Perplexed.* Chicago: University of Chicago Press; 2008.

87. Bhikkhu T. *Iddhipada-vibhanga Sutta: Analysis of the Bases of Power* (SN 51.20), translated from the Pali 2010; http://www.accesstoinsight.org/tipitaka /sn/sn51/sn51.020.than.html, accessed March 24, 2012.

88. Houshmand Z, Livingston RB, Wallace BA, eds. *Consciousness at the Crossroads: Conversations with the Dalai Lama on Brain Science and Buddhism.* Ithaca, NY: Snow Lion Publications; 1999.

89. Tucker JB. Children's reports of past-life memories: A review. *Explore.* 2008;4(4):244-248.

90. Gardner R. Miracles of healing in Anglo-Celtic Northumbria as recorded by the Venerable Bede and his contemporaries: A reappraisal in the light of twentieth century experience. *Brit Med J.* 1983;287(24-31):1927-1933.

91. O'Regan B, Hirshberg C. *Spontaneous Remission: An Annotated Bibliography.* Sausalito, CA: Institute of Noetic Sciences; 1993.

92. Aziz MA. *Religion and Mysticism in Early Islam: Theology and Sufism in Yemen.* London and New York: I.B. Tauris, 2011.

93. Hoffman E. *The Way of Splendor: Jewish Mysticism and Modern Psychology.* 25th ed. Lanham, MD: Rowman & Littlefield; 2007.

94. Kaplan A. *Jewish Meditation: A Practical Guide.* New York: Schocken Books; 1985.

95. Cleary T. *The Flower Ornament Scripture: A Translation of the Avatamsaka Sutra.* Boston and London: Shambala; 1993.

96. Summers M. *The Physical Phenomena of Mysticism: With Especial References to the Stigmata, Divine and Diabolic.* London: Rider & Company; 1950.

97. Grosso M. *The Strange Case of Saint Joseph Cupertino: Ecstasy and the Mind-Body Problem.* New York: Oxford University Press; 2013.

98. Lamont P. *The First Psychic: The Peculiar Mystery of a Notorious Victorian Wizard.* London: Abacus; 2005.

99. Leuba JH. *The Psychology of Religious Mysticism* (revised ed.). New York: Harcourt, Brace; 1929.

100. Hof W, Rosales J. *Becoming the Iceman: Pushing Past Perceived Limits*. Minneapolis: Mill City Press; 2012.

101. International Association of Universities. 2012; http://www.iau-aiu .net/content/list-heis, accessed February 11, 2012.

102. Hill A. *Paranormal Media: Audiences, Spirits and Magic in Popular Culture*. Florence, KY: Routledge; 2010.

103. Kripal JJ. *Mutants and Mystics: Science Fiction, Superhero Comics, and the Paranormal*. Chicago: University of Chicago Press; 2011.

104. Adityanjee, Raju GS, Khandelwal SK. Current status of multiple personality disorder in India. *Am J Psychiat*. 1989;146(12):1607-1610.

105. Bliss EL, Jeppsen EA. Prevalence of multiple personality among inpatients and outpatients. *Am J Psychiat*. 1985;142(2):250-251.

106. Baumeister RF, Masicampo EJ, DeWall CN. Prosocial benefits of feeling free: Disbelief in free will increases aggression and reduces helpfulness. *Pers Soc Psychol Bull*. 2009;35:260.

107. Sahdra BK, MacLean KA, Ferrer E, et al. Enhanced response inhibition during intensive meditation training predicts improvements in self-reported adaptive socioemotional functioning. *Emotion*. 2011;11(2):299–312.

108. Eddington SAS. *Science and the Unseen World (Swarthmore Lecture)*. New York: Macmillan; 1929.

109. Josephson B. Personal communication, 2012.

110. McLean CP, Miller NA. Changes in critical thinking skills following a course on science and pseudoscience: A quasi-experimental study. *Teach Psychol*. 2010;37:85-90.

111. Radin DI, Machado F, Zangari W. Effects of distant healing intention through time and space: Two exploratory studies. *Subtle Energies and Energy Med*. 2000;11(3):207-240.

112. Banziger G. Normalizing the paranormal: Short-term and long-term change in belief in the paranormal among older learners during a short course. *Teach Psychol*. 1983;10(3):212-214.

113. Sharps MJ, Matthews J, Asten J. Cognition and belief in paranormal phenomena: Gestalt/feature-intensive processing theory and tendencies toward ADHD, depression, and dissociation. *J Psychol*. 2006;140(6):579-590.

114. Francis LJ, Williams E, Robbins M. Personality, conventional Christian belief and unconventional paranormal belief: A study among teenagers. *Brit J Relig Educ*. 2010;32(1):31-39.

115. Blagrove M, French CC, Jones G. Probabilistic reasoning, affirmative bias and belief in precognitive dreams. *Appl Cognitive Psychol*. 2006;20:65-83.

WORKS CITED

116. Roe CA. Critical thinking and belief in the paranormal: A re-evaluation. *Brit J Psychol*. 1999;90:85-98.

117. Manza L, Hilperts K, Hindley L, Marco C, Santana A, Hawk MV. Exposure to science is not enough: The influence of classroom experiences on belief in paranormal phenomena. *Teach Psychol*. 2010;37:165–171.

118. Stanovich KE. *How to Think Straight About Psychology*. 9th ed. Boston: Allyn and Bacon, Pearson Education; 2010.

119. Broad W, Wade N. *Betrayers of the Truth: Fraud and Deceit in the Halls of Science*. New York: Simon & Schuster; 1982.

120. Wiseman R. *Paranormality: Why We See What Isn't There*. London: Spin Solutions; 2011.

121. Swami V, Pietschnig J, Stieger S, Voracek M. Alien psychology: Associations between extraterrestrial beliefs and paranormal ideation, superstitious beliefs, schizotypy, and the Big Five personality factors. *Appl Cogn Psychol*. 2011;25:647-653.

122. Musch J, Ehrenberg K. Probability misjudgment, cognitive ability, and belief in the paranormal. *Brit J Psychol*. 2002;93(169-177).

123. Broad CD. The relevance of psychical research to philosophy. *Philosophy*. 1949;24:291-309.

124. Begley S. Belief in the paranormal reflects normal brain activity carried to an extreme. *Newsweek*. November 3, 2008.

125. Shermer M. *The Believing Brain: From Ghosts and Gods to Politics and Conspiracies—How We Construct Beliefs and Reinforce Them as Truths*. New York: Times Books; 2011.

126. Sheldrake R. *Dogs That Know When Their Owners Are Coming Home*. Updated rev. ed. New York: Three Rivers Press; 2011.

127. Radin D. A dog that seems to know when his owner is coming home: Effect of environmental variables. *J Sci Explor*. 2002;16(4):579-592.

128. Penman D. Could there be proof to the theory that we're ALL psychic? 2008; http://www.dailymail.co.uk/news/article-510762/Could-proof-theory-ALL-psychic.html, accessed February 17, 2012.

129. Investigations S. Professional materalistic debunkers' concessions on the evidence for psi phenomena and psi research; http://www.skepticalinvestigations.org/Examskeptics/Concessions_debunkers.html, accessed February 17, 2012.

130. Mason R. Bringing Sufi rapid healing methods into the laboratory. *Altern Complem Ther*. 2004(April):90-94.

131. Dyson F. One in a million. *New York Times Review of Books*. March 25, 2004.

132. Shermer M. Miracle on probability street. *Scientific American*. July 26, 2004.

133. Horgan J. Freeman Dyson, global warming, ESP and the fun of being "bunkrapt." *Cross-Check. Sci Am.* 2011;2012.

134. Schiltz M, Wiseman R, Watt C, Radin DI. Of two minds: Skeptic-proponent collaboration within parapsychology. *Brit J Psychol.* 2006;97:313-322.

135. Schmeidler G, Murphy G. The influence of belief and disbelief in ESP upon individual scoring levels. *J Exp Psychol.* 1946;36(3):271-276.

136. Lawrence T. Bringing in the sheep: A meta-analysis of sheep/goat experiments. Paper presented at: Parapsychological Association Annual Conference, 1993; Toronto, Canada.

137. Thalbourne MA. Relation between transliminality and openness to experience. *Psychol Rep.* June 2000;86(3, Pt 1):909-910.

138. Arcangel D. *Afterlife Encounters: Ordinary People, Extraordinary Experiences.* Charlottesville, VA: Hampton Roads; 2005.

139. Kennedy JE. Personality and motivations to believe, misbelieve, and disbelieve in paranormal phenomena. *J Parapsychol.* 2005;69:263-292.

140. Deacon TW. *Incomplete Nature: How Mind Emerged from Matter.* New York: Norton; 2011.

141. Tart CT. *The End of Materialism: How Evidence of the Paranormal Is Bringing Science and Spirit Together.* Oakland, CA: New Harbinger Publications/Noetic Books; 2009.

142. Sheldrake R. *Science Set Free.* New York: Crown Publishing; 2012.

143. Noë A. *Out of Our Heads: Why You Are Not Your Brain, and Other Lessons from the Biology of Consciousness.* New York: Hill and Wang; 2010.

144. Lanza R, Berman B. *Biocentrism: How Life and Consciousness Are the Keys to Understanding the True Nature of the Universe* Dallas: BenBella Books; 2010.

145. Rama S. *Living with the Himalayan Masters.* Honesdale, PA: Himalayan Institute Press; 2007.

146. Paranjape ME, Lama DF, eds. *Science, Spirituality and the Modernisation of India.* London, UK: Anthem Press India; 2009.

147. Aharonov Y, Anandan J, Maclay GJ, Suzuki J. Model for entangled states with spin-spin interaction. *Phys Rev A.* 2004;70(052114).

148. Christensen A. General yoga information; http://www.americanyogaassociation.org/general.html, accessed January 14, 2012.

149. Fontana D. *The Meditator's Handbook: A Comprehensive Guide to Eastern and Western Meditation Techniques.* Rockport, MA: Element; 1992.

150. Shankman R. *The Experience of Samadhi: An In-Depth Exploration of Buddhist Meditation.* Boston and London: Shambhala; 2008.

151. Ott U. The role of absorption for the study of yoga. *J Meditation and Meditation Res.* 2003;3:21-26.

152. Forman RKC. *Enlightenment Ain't What It's Cracked Up to Be: A Journey of Discovery, Snow and Jazz in the Soul.* Alresford, Hants, UK: O-Books, John Hunt Publishing; 2011.

153. Helrich CS. Is there a basis for teleology in physics? *Zygon.* 2007;42(1):97-110.

154. Ma X-s, Zotter S, Kofler J, et al. Experimental delayed-choice entanglement swapping. *Nat Phys.* 2012;advance online publication.

155. Aharanov Y, Tollaksen J. New insights on time-symmetry in quantum mechanics. In: Chiao RY, Cohen ML, Leggett AJ, Phillips WD, Harper CL, eds. *Visions of Discovery: New Light on Physics, Cosmology, and Consciousness.* Cambridge, UK: Cambridge University Press; 2007.

156. Merali Z. Back from the future. 2010; http://discovermagazine .com/2010/apr/01-back-from-the-future/article_view?b_start:int=0&-C=, accessed March 3, 2012.

157. Verschuur GL. *Hidden Attraction: The History and Mystery of Magnetism.* Oxford, UK: Oxford University Press; 1993.

158. Benson H, Lehmann JW, Malhotra M, Goldman RF, Hopkins J, Epstein MD. Body temperature changes during the practice of g Tum-mo yoga. *Nature.* 1982;295:234-236.

159. Pickkers P. The effects of concentration/meditation on the innate immune response during human endotoxemia. 2011; http://clinicaltrials.gov /ct2/show/NCT01352871, accessed March 24, 2012.

160. ScienceDaily. Research on "Iceman" Wim Hof suggests it may be possible to influence autonomic nervous system and immune response. April 22, 2011; http://www.sciencedaily.com/releases/2011/04/110422090203.htm, accessed February 18, 2012.

161. Scientists baffled by Prahlad Jani, man who doesn't eat or drink. 2012; http://abcnews.go.com/Health/International/man-eat-drink /story?id=10787036, accessed April 1, 2012.

162. Werner M, Stockli T. *Life from Light: Is It Possible to Live Without Food?* Forest Row, UK: Clairview Books; 2007.

163. Braud WG. Patañjali yoga and siddhis: Their relevance to parapsychological theory and research. In: K. Ramakrishna Rao, Anand C. Paranjpe, Ajit K. Dalal, eds. *Handbook of Indian Psychology,* Cambridge, UK: Foundation Books; 2008: 217-243.

164. Bobrow RS. Paranormal phenomena in the medical literature sufficient smoke to warrant a search for fire. *Med Hypotheses.* June 2003;60(6):864-868.

165. Azuma N, Stevenson I. "Psychic surgery" in the Philippines as a form of group hypnosis. *Am J Clin Hypn.* July 1988;31(1):61-67.

166. Storm L, Tressoldi PE, Di Risio L. Meta-analysis of free-response studies, 1992–2008: Assessing the noise reduction model in parapsychology. *Psychol Bull.* July 2010;136(4):471-485.

167. Braud WG. Psi conducive conditions: Explorations and interpretations. In: Shapin B, Coly L, eds. *Psi and States of Awareness.* New York: Parapsychology Foundation; 1978.

168. Honorton C. Psi and internal attention states. In: Wolman BB, ed. *Handbook of Parapsychology.* New York: Van Nostrand Rheinhold; 1977:435-472.

169. Roney-Dougal SM, Solfvin J, Fox J. An exploration of the degree of meditation attainment in relation to psychic awareness with Tibetan Buddhists. *J Sci Explor.* 2008;22(2):161-178.

170. Roney-Dougal SM, Solfvin J. Exploring the relationship between Tibetan meditation attainment and precognition. *J Sci Explor.* 2011;25(1):29-46.

171. Crick F. *The Astonishing Hypothesis: The Scientific Search for the Soul.* New York: Touchstone; 1994.

172. LeShan L. Henry Margenau quote. *The Science of the Paranormal: The Last Frontier.* Northamptonshire, UK: Aquarian Press; 1987:118.

173. Dossey L. *The Power of Premonitions.* New York: Dutton Adult; 2009.

174. Wiseman R, Watt C. Belief in psychic ability and the misattribution hypothesis: A qualitative review. *Brit J Psychol.* August 2006;97(Pt 3):323-338.

175. Pratt JG, Rhine JB. *Extra-Sensory Perception After Sixty Years: A Critical Appraisal of the Research in Extra-Sensory Perception.* Boston: Bruce Humphries; 1967.

176. Honorton C. Meta-analysis of psi ganzfeld research: A response to Hyman. *J Parapsychol.* 1985;49:51-92.

177. Honorton C, Ferrari DC. "Future telling": A meta-analysis of forced-choice precognition experiments, 1935–1987. *J Parapsychol.* 1989;53:281-308.

178. Rosenthal R, Rosnow RL. *Essentials of Behavioral Research.* 3rd ed. New York: McGraw-Hill; 2008.

179. Richard FD, Bond CF Jr. , Stokes-Zoota JJ. One hundred years of social psychology quantitatively described. *Rev Gen Psychol.* 2003;7:331-363.

180. Jahn RG, Dunne BJ. *Margins of Reality.* New York: Jovanovich; 1987.

181. Utts J. An assessment of the evidence for psychic functioning. *J Sci Explor.* 1996;10(1):3-30.

182. Dunne BJ, Jahn RG. Information and uncertainty in remote perception research. *J Sci Explor.* 2003;17(2):207-241.

183. Krippner S, Honorton C, Ullman M. An experiment in dream telepathy with "The Grateful Dead." *J Am Soc Psychosom Dent Med.* 1973;20(1):9-17.

184. Radin DI. Unconscious perception of future emotions: An experiment in presentiment. *J Sci Explor.* 1997;11:163-180.

185. Radin DI. Electrodermal presentiments of future emotions. *J Sci Explor.* 2004;18:253-274.

186. Tressoldi P, Martinelli M, Massaccesi S, Sartori L. Heart rate differences between targets and non-targets in intuitive tasks. *Hum Physiol.* 2005;31(6):646-650.

187. McCraty R, Atkinson M, Bradley RT. Electrophysiological evidence of intuition: Part 1. The surprising role of the heart. *J Altern Complem Med.* 2004;10:133-143.

188. Radin D, Borges A. Intuition through time: What does the seer see? *Explore.* 2009;5:200-211.

189. Radin D, Lobach E. Toward understanding the placebo effect: Investigating a possible retrocausal factor. *J Altern Complem Med.* 2007;13(7):733-739.

190. Bierman DJ, Scholte HS. A fMRI brain imaging study of presentiment. *J Int Soc Life Info Sci.* 2002;20(2):380-388.

191. Sequeira H, Hot P, Silvert L, Delplanque S. Electrical autonomic correlates of emotion. *Int J Psychophysiol.* January 2009;71(1):50-56.

192. Bradley MM, Lang PJ. The International Affective Picture System (IAPS) in the study of emotion and attention. In: Coan JA, Allen JJB, eds. *Handbook of Emotion Elicitation and Assessment.* New York: Cambridge University Press; 2007.

193. Gross CG. The fire that comes from the eye. *Neuroscientist.* 1999;5:58-64.

194. Schmidt S, Scheider R, Utts J, Walach H. Distant intentionality and the feeling of being stared at: Two meta-analyses. *Brit J Psychol.* 2004;95:235.

195. Radin DI. The sense of being stared at: A preliminary meta-analysis. *J Conscious Studies.* 2005;12(6):95-100.

196. Bosch H, Steinkamp F, Boller E. Examining psychokinesis: The interaction of human intention with random number generators—a meta-analysis. *Psychol Bull.* 2006;132(4):497.

197. Radin D, Nelson R, Dobyns Y, Houtkooper J. Reexamining psychokinesis: Commentary on the Bösch, Steinkamp and Boller meta-analysis. *Psychol Bull.* 2006:529-532.

198. Titelman GY. *Random House Dictionary of Popular Proverbs and Sayings.* New York: Random House; 1996.

199. Steinhauer SR, Hakerem G. The pupillary response in cognitive psychophysiology and schizophrenia. In: Friedman D, Bruder G, eds. *Psychophysiology and Experimental Psychopathology: A Tribute to Samuel Sutton.* Vol 658. New York: Annals of the New York Academy of Sciences; 1992:182-204.

200. Bitsios P, Szabadi E, Bradshaw CM. The fear-inhibited light reflex: Importance of the anticipation of an aversive event. *Int J Psychophysiol.* 2004; 52:87-95.

201. Loewenfeld IE. *The Pupil: Anatomy, Physiology, and Clinical Applications.* Ames: Iowa State University Press; 1993.

202. Laeng B, Teodorescu D-S. Eye scanpaths during visual imagery reenact those of perception of the same visual scene. *Cognitive Sci.* 2002;26:207-231.

203. Andreassi JL. Pupillary response and behavior. *Psychophysiology: Human Behavior and Physiological Response.* Mahwah, NJ: Lawrence Erlbaum; 2000:218-233.

204. Bacher LF, Smotherman WP. Spontaneous eye blinking in human infants: A review. *Dev Psychobiol.* 2004;44:95-102.

205. Good IJ. Letter to the editor. *J Parapsychol.* 1961;25:58.

206. van Boxtel GJM, Böcker KBE. Cortical measures of anticipation. *J Psychophysiol.* 2004;18:61-76.

207. McCraty R, Atkinson M, Bradley RT. Electrophysiological evidence of intuition: Part 2. A system-wide process? *J Altern Complem Med.* 2004;10:325-336.

208. Cahn R, Polich J. Meditation states and traits: EEG, ERP, and neuroimaging studies. *Psychol Bull.* 2006;132:180-211.

209. Newberg A, Alavi A, Baime M, Pourdehnad M, Santanna J, d'Aquili E. The measurement of regional cerebral blood flow during the complex cognitive task of meditation: A preliminary psychiatry research study. *Neuroimaging.* 2001;106(2):113-122.

210. Josipovic Z. Duality and nonduality in meditation research. *Conscious Cogn.* 2010;19:1119-1121.

211. Wittmann M, van Wassenhove V, Craig AD, Paulus MP. The neural substrates of subjective time dilation. *Front Human Neurosci.* 2010;4:1-9.

212. Woods JH. *The Yoga System of Patanjali.* Cambridge, MA: Harvard University Press; 1927.

213. Woods JH. *The Yoga System of Patanjal.* Delhi: Motilal Banarsidass; 2007.

214. Hartman BO, Secrist GE. Situational awareness is more than exceptional vision. *Aviat Space Envir Med*. 1991;62:1084-1089.

215. Rosen R. *Anticipatory Systems*. New York: Pergamon Press; 1985.

216. Eagleman DM, Sejnowski T. Motion integration and postdiction in visual awareness. *Science*. 2000;287:2036-2038.

217. Wolf FA. The timing of conscious experience: A causality-violating, two-valued, transactional interpretation of subjective antedating and spatial-temporal projection. *J Sci Explor*. 1998;12:511-542.

218. Dennett DC. Temporal anomalies of consciousness. In: Christen Y, Churchland PS, eds. *Neurophilosophy and Alzheimer's Disease*. Berlin: Springer-Verlag; 1992.

219. Libet B. Unconscious cerebral initiative and the role of conscious will in voluntary action. *Behav Brain Sci*. 1985;8:529-566.

220. Radin DI, Vieten C, Michel L, Delorme A. Electrocortical activity prior to unpredictable stimuli in meditators and non-meditators. *Explore*. 2011;7:286-299.

221. Radin D, Vieten C, Michel L, Delorme A. Electrocortical activity prior to unpredictable stimuli in meditators and non-meditators. *Explore*. In press.

222. Mossbridge J, Tressoldi P, Utts J. Predictive anticipatory activity preceding unpredictable stimuli: A meta-analysis. *Front Percep Sci*. 2012;3:1-18.

223. Yagi Y, Ikoma S, Kikuchi T. Attentional modulation of the mere exposure effect. *J Exp Psychol Learn Mem Cogn*. November 2009;35(6):1403-1410.

224. Bem DJ. Feeling the future: Experimental evidence for anomalous retroactive influences on cognition and affect. *J Pers Soc Psychol*. 2011;100(3):407-425.

225. Bem DJ, Utts J, Johnson WO. Must psychologists change the way they analyze their data? *J Pers Soc Psychol*. 2011;101(4):716-719.

226. Camp BH. Statement in notes section. *J Parapsychol*. 1937;1:305.

227. Miller G. ESP paper rekindles discussion about statistics. *Science*. January 21, 2011:331.

228. Holmes B. ESP evidence airs science's dirty laundry. *New Scientist*. January 11, 2012.

229. LeBel E, Peters K. Fearing the future of empirical psychology: Bem's evidence of psi as a case study of deficiencies in modal research practice. *Rev Gen Psychol*. 2011;15(4):371-379.

230. Wagenmakers EJ, Wetzels R, Borsboom D, van der Maas H. Why psychologists must change the way they analyze their data: The case of psi. *J Pers Soc Psychol*. 2011;100:426-432.

231. Galak J, LeBoeuf RA, Nelson LD, Simmons JP. Correcting the past: Failures to replicate psi. *J Pers Soc Psychol*. Forthcoming (June 19, 2012).

232. Tributsch H. The bionic anticipation of natural disasters. *J Bionic Eng*. 2005;2(3):123-144.

233. Wildey C. *Impulse Response of Biological Systems*. Arlington, TX: Department of Electrical Engineering, University of Texas; 2001.

234. Alvarez F. Anticipatory alarm behavior in Bengalese finches. *J Sci Explor*. 2010;24(4):599-610.

235. Alvarez F. Higher anticipatory response at 13.5 ± 1 h local sidereal time in Zebra finches. *J Parapsychol*. 2010;72(2):323-334.

236. Radin DI. Predicting the unpredictable: 75 years of experimental evidence. In: Sheehan DP, ed. *Quantum Retrocausation: Theory and Experiment*. Melville, NY: American Institute of Physics; 2011.

237. Sheehan DP. Frontiers of time: Retrocausation experiment and theory. *AIP Conference Proceedings 863*. Melville, NY: American Institute of Physics; 2006.

238. Twain M. Mental telegraphy. A manuscript with a history. *Harper's New Monthly Magazine*. Vol 84. 1891:95-104.

239. Wackermann J, Putz P, Allefeld C. Ganzfeld-induced hallucinatory experience, its phenomenology and cerebral electrophysiology. *Cortex*. November-December 2008;44(10):1364-1378.

240. Delgado-Romero EA, Howard GS. Finding and correcting flawed research literatures. *Humanistic Psychol*. 2005;33(4):293-303.

241. Milton J, Wiseman R. Does psi exist? Lack of replication of an anomalous process of information transfer. *Psychol Bull*. 1999;125:387-391.

242. Goldbert C. Brain scan tests fail to support validity of ESP. *Boston Globe*, January 14, 2008: C1.

243. Moulton ST, Kosslyn SM. Using neuroimaging to resolve the psi debate. *J Cogn Neurosci*. January 2008;20(1):182-192.

244. Standish LJ, Johnson LC, Kozak L, Richards T. Evidence of correlated functional magnetic resonance imaging signals between distant human brains. *Altern Ther*. 2003;9:122-125.

245. Richards TL, Kozak L, Johnson LC, Standish LJ. Replicable functional magnetic resonance imaging. evidence of correlated brain signals between physically and sensory isolated subjects. *J Altern Complem Med*. 2005;11(6):955-963.

246. Achterberg J, Cooke K, Richards T, Standish LJ, Kozak L. Evidence for correlations between distant intentionality and brain function in recipients:

A functional magnetic resonance imaging analysis. *J Altern Complem Med.* 2005;11(6):965-971.

247. Venkatasubramanian G, Jayakumar PN, Nagendra HR, Nagaraja D, Deeptha R, Gangadhar BN. Investigating paranormal phenomena: Functional brain imaging of telepathy. *Int J Yoga.* July 2008;1(2):66-71.

248. Bierman D. Presentiment in a fMRI experiment with meditators. *Euro-Parapsychological Association Convention.* Paris, October 28, 2007.

249. Bem DJ, Honorton C. Does psi exist? Replicable evidence for an anomalous process of information transfer. *Psychol Bull.* 1994;115:4-18.

250. Storm L, Ertel S. Does psi exist? Comments on Milton and Wiseman's (1999) meta-analysis of ganzfeld research. *Psychol Bull.* 2001;127:424-433.

251. Bem DJ, Palmer J, Broughton RS. Updating the ganzfeld database: A victim of its own success? *J Parapsychol.* 2001;65:207-218.

252. Hyman R. The ganzfeld psi experiment: A critical appraisal. *J Parapsychol.* 1985;49:3-49.

253. Tressoldi PE. Extraordinary claims require extraordinary evidence: The case of non-local perception, a classical and Bayesian review of evidences. *Front Psychol.* 2011;2.

254. Jeffreys H. *The Theory of Probability,* 3rd ed. Oxford, UK: Oxford University Press; 1961.

255. Milton J. Meta-analysis of free-response ESP studies without altered states of consciousness. *J Parapsychol.* 1997;61:279-319.

256. Sheldrake R, Smart P. Experimental tests for telephone telepathy. *J Soc Psych Res.* 2003;67:184-199.

257. Sheldrake R, Smart P. Videotaped experiments on telephone telepathy. *J Parapsychol.* 2003;67:187-206.

258. Sheldrake R, Avraamides L, Novak M. Sensing the sending of SMS messages: An automated test. *Explore: J Sci Heal.* 2009;5:272-276.

259. Sheldrake R, Avraamides L. An automated test for telepathy in connection with emails. *J Sci Explor.* 2009;23(1):29-36.

260. Sheldrake R, Lambert M. An automated online telepathy test. *J Sci Explor.* 2007;21:511-522.

261. Sheldrake R, Beharee A. A rapid online telepathy test. *Psychol Rep.* 2009;104:957-970.

262. Pearson C. *The Complete Book of Yogic Flying.* Fairfield, IA: Maharishi Unviersity of Management Press; 2008.

263. Hagelin JS, Orme-Johnson DW, Rainforth M, Cavanaugh K, Alexander CN. Results of the National Demonstration Project to reduce violent crime

and improve governmental effectiveness in Washington, D.C. *Soc Indic Res.* 1999;47:153-201.

264. Lama D, Ekman P. *Emotional Awareness: Overcoming the Obstacles to Psychological Balance and Compassion.* New York: Times Books; 2008.

265. Radin DI, Stone J, Levine E, et al. Compassionate intention as a therapeutic intervention by partners of cancer patients: Effects of distant intention on the patients' autonomic nervous system. *Explore: J Sci Heal.* 2008;4(4):235-243.

266. Barnes P, Powell-Griner E, McFann K, Nahin R. Complementary and alternative medicine use among adults: United States. *CDC Advance Data Report #343.* May 27, 2004.

267. Canda ER, Furman LD. *Spiritual Diversity in Social Work Practice: The Heart of Helping.* New York: Free Press; 1999.

268. Mao JJ, Farrar J T, Xie S X, Bowman, M A, Armstrong K. Use of complementary and alternative medicine and prayer among a national sample of cancer survivors compared to other populations without cancer. *Complement Ther Med.* 2007;15(1):21-29.

269. Wachholtz A, Sambamoorthi U. National trends in prayer use as a coping mechanism for health concerns: Changes from 2002 to 2007. *Psychol Rel Spirit.* 2011;3(2):67-77.

270. Sloan RP, Ramakrishnan R. The MANTRA II study. *The Lancet.* 2005;366:1769-1770.

271. Walach H. Generalized entanglement: A new theoretical model for understanding the effects of complementary and alternative medicine. *J Alt Comp Med.* 2005;11(3):549-559.

272. Astin JA, Harkness E, Ernst E. The efficacy of "distant healing": A systematic review of randomized trials. *Ann Intern Med.* 2000;132:903-910.

273. Hodge DR. Social justice and people of faith: A transnational prespective. *Social Work.* 2007;52(2):139-148.

274. Cha KYW, D. P. Does prayer influence the success of in vitro fertilization-embryo transfer? Report of a masked, randomized trial. *J Reprod Med.* 2001;46(9):781-787.

275. Masters KS, and Spielmans G I. Prayer and health: Review, meta-analysis, and research agenda. *J Beh Med.* 2007;30(4):329-338.

276. Roberts L, Ahmed I, Hall S, Davison A. Intercessory prayer for the alleviation of ill health. *Cochrane Data System Rev.* 2011(3):1-48.

277. Schmidt S. The attention focusing facilitation paradigm: Remote helping for meditation? A meta-analysis. Paper presented at: Parapsychological Association Annual Convention, 2010; Paris.

278. Shen D. Unexpected behavior of matter in conjunction with human consciousness. *J Sci Explor*. 2010;24(1):41-52.

279. Wu B, Zhou L, Luo X. *Introduction to the Science of the Human Body [Chinese]*. Cheng Du, China: Si Chuan University Press; 1998.

280. Farwell L. *How Consciousness Commands Matter: The New Scientific Revolution and the Evidence That Anything Is Possible*. Fairfield, IA: Sunstar Publishing; 1999.

281. Farwell LA, Farwell GW. Quantum-mechanical processes and consciousness. *Bull Am Physical Soc*. 1995;40(2):956-957.

282. Beloff J, Evans L. A radioactivity test of psycho-kinesis. *J Soc Psych Res*. 1961;41:41-46.

283. Schub MH. A critique of the parapsychological random number generator meta-analyses of Radin and Nelson. *J Sci Explor*. 2006;20:402-419.

284. Radin DI, Nelson RD, Dobyns YH, Houtkooper J. Assessing the evidence for mind-matter interaction effects. *J Sci Explor*. 2006;30(3):361-374.

285. Collins HH. *Changing Order: Replication and Induction in Scientific Practice*. Beverly Hills, CA: Sage; 1985.

286. Nelson RD, Radin DI, Shoup R, Bancel P. Correlation of continuous random data with major world events. *Found Phys Lett*. 2002;15(6):537-550.

287. Nelson RD, Jahn RG, Dunne BJ, Dobyns YH, Bradish GJ. FieldREG II: Consciousness field effects: Replications and explorations. *J Sci Explor*. 1998;12(3):425-454.

288. Radin DI. Exploring relationships between random physical events and mass human attention: Asking for whom the bell tolls. *J Sci Explor*. 2002;16(4):533-548.

289. Nelson RD, Jahn RG, Dunne BJ, Dobyns YH, Bradish GJ. FieldREGII: Consciousness field effects: Replications and explorations. *Explore*. 2007;3(3):279-293.

290. Atwater FH. Accessing anomalous states of consciousness with a binaural beat technology. *J Sci Explor*. 1997;11(3):263-274.

291. Brady B, Stevens L. Binaural-beat induced theta EEG activity and hypnotic susceptibility. *Am J Clin Hypn*. July 2000;43(1):53-69.

292. Wahbeh H, Calabrese C, Zwickey H. Binaural beat technology in humans: A pilot study to assess psychologic and physiologic effects. *J Altern Complem Med*. January-February 2007;13(1):25-32.

293. Radin D, Atwater FH. Exploratory evidence for correlations between entrained mental coherence and random physical systems. *J Sci Explor*. 2009;23(3):263-272.

294. Nelson R, Bancel P. Effects of mass consciousness: Changes in random data during global events. *Explore: J Sci Heal*. 2011;7(6):373-383.

295. Houtkooper J. Arguing for an observational theory of paranormal phenomena. *J Sci Explor.* 2002;16(2):171.

296. Feynman RP, Leighton RB, Sands M. *The Feynman Lectures on Physics.* Vol 3. New York: Addison-Wesley; 1965.

297. Juffmann T, Milic A, Müllneritsch M, et al. Real-time single-molecule imaging of quantum interference. *Nat Nanotech.* 2012.

298. Jammer, M. *The Philosophy of Quantum Mechanics.* Wiley: New York; 1974.

299. D'Espagnat B. The quantum theory and reality. *Scientific American.* 1979:158.

300. Neumann JV. *Mathematical Foundations of Quantum Mechanics.* Princeton, NJ: Princeton University Press; 1955.

301. Stapp H. *Mindful Universe: Quantum Mechanics and the Participating Observer.* New York: Springer; 2007.

302. Squires EJ. Many views of one world—an interpretation of quantum theory. *Eur J Physics.* 1987;8(3):171.

303. Goldstein S. Quantum theory without observers, I and II. *Physics Today.* 1998:38.

304. Fuchs C, Peres A. Quantum theory needs no "interpretation." *Physics Today.* 2000;53(3):70.

305. Bell JS. *Speakable and Unspeakable in Quantum Mechanics.* Cambridge, UK: Cambridge University Press; 1987.

306. Zeilinger A. Experiment and the foundations of quantum physics. *Rev Mod Physics.* 1999;71:288-298.

307. d'Espagnat B. Consciousness and the Wigner's friend problem. *Found Physics,* 2005;35(12):1943.

308. Rosenblum B, Kuttner F. *Quantum Enigma: Physics Encounters Consciousness.* Oxford: Oxford University Press; 2006.

309. Bub J. *Interpreting the Quantum World.* Cambridge, UK: Cambridge University Press; 1997.

310. Rosenblum B, Kuttner F. The observer in the quantum experiment. *Found Physics.* 2002;32(8):1273.

311. Johnson G. Here they are, science's 10 most beautiful experiments. 2002, September 24; http://www.nytimes.com/2002/09/24/science/here-they-are-science-s-10-most-beautiful-experiments.html?pagewanted=all&src=pm.

312. TeachSpin I. Two-slit interference, one photon as a time. 2012; http://www.teachspin.com/instruments/two_slit/index.shtml.

313. Tittel W, Brendel J, Gisin B, Herzog T, Zbinden H, Gisin N. Experimental demonstration of quantum correlations over more than 10 km. *Phys Rev A.* 1998;57:3229.

314. Freire O Jr. Quantum dissidents: Research on the foundations of quantum theory circa 1970. *Stud Hist Philos Sci Part B: Stud Hist Philos Mod Physics*. 2009;40(4):280.

315. Radin D, Nelson R. Evidence for consciousness-related anomalies in random physical systems. *Found Physics*. 1989;19:1499.

316. Schmidt H. PK tests with pre-recorded and pre-inspected seed numbers. *J Parapsychol*. 1981;45:87.

317. Hall J, Kim C, McElroy B, Shimony A. Wave-packet reduction as a medium of communication. *Found Physics*. 1977;7:759-767.

318. Bierman DJ. Does consciousness collapse the wave-packet? *Mind and Matter*. 2003;2:45-58.

319. Jahn G. The persistent paradox of psychic phenomena: An engineering perspective. *Proc of the IEEE*. 1982;70:136.

320. Ibison M, Jeffers S. A double-slit diffraction experiment to investigate claims of consciousness-related anomalies. *J Sci Explor*. 1998;12:543.

321. Jeffers S, Sloan J. A low light level diffraction experiments for anomalies research. *J Sci Explor*. 1992;6:333.

322. Radin DI. Testing nonlocal observation as a source of intuitive knowledge. *Explore: J Sci Heal*. 2008;4(1):23-35.

323. Radin DI, Michel L, Galdamez K, Wendland P, Rickenbach R, Delorme A. Consciousness and the double-slit interference pattern: Six experiments. *Physics Essays*. 2012;25(2):157-171.

324. Kim YH, Yu R, Kulik SP, Shih Y, Scully MO. Delayed "Choice" quantum eraser. *Phys Rev Lett*. January 3, 2000;84(1):1-5.

325. Tellegen A, Atkinson G. Openness to absorbing and self-altering experiences ("absorption"), a trait related to hypnotic susceptibility. *J Abnorm Psychol*. 1974;83:268.

326. Schmeidler G, Murphy G. The influence of belief and disbelief in ESP upon individual scoring levels. *J Abnor Psychol*. 1946;83:268.

327. McMoneagle J. *The Stargate Chronicles: Memoirs of a Psychic Spy*. Charlottesville, VA: Hampton Roads Pub.; 2002.

328. Smith PH. *Reading the Enemy's Mind : Inside Star Gate, America's Psychic Espionage Program*. New York: Tom Doherty Associates; 2005.

329. Targ R. *The Reality of ESP*. Wheaton, IL: Quest Books; 2012.

330. Phillips SM. *Extra-Sensory Perception of Quarks*. Wheaton, IL: Quest Books; 1980.

331. Phillips SM. Extrasensory perception of subatomic particles I. Historical evidence. *J Sci Explor*. 1995;9(4):489-525.

332. Atwater FH. *Captain of My Ship, Master of My Soul: Living with Guidance.* Charlottesville, VA: Hampton Roads Pub.; 2001.

333. Graff DE. *Tracks in the Psychic Wilderness: An Exploration of ESP, Remote Viewing, Precognitive Dreaming and Synchronicity.* London: Vega; 2003.

334. Mayer EL. *Extraordinary Knowing: Science, Skepticism, and the Inexplicable Powers of the Human Mind.* New York: Bantam Books; 2007.

335. Kripal JJ. *Authors of the Impossible: The Paranormal and the Sacred.* Chicago:: University of Chicago Press; 2010.

336. Schmeidler G. High ESP scores after a swami's brief instruction in meditation and breathing. *J Amer Soc Psych Res.* 1970;64:100-103.

337. Schmeidler G. ESP experiments 1978–1992. In: Krippner S, ed. *Advances in Parapsychological Research.* Vol 7. Jefferson, NC: McFarland; 1994:104-197.

338. Rao KR. *Cognitive Anomalies, Consciousness and Yoga.* Vol XVI, Part 1. New Delhi: Matrix Publishers; 2011.

339. Roney-Dougal SM. Taboo and belief in Tibetan psychic tradition. *J Soc Psych Res.* 2006;70.4(885):193-210.

340. Roney-Dougal SM, Solfvin J. Yogic attainment in relation to awareness of precognitive targets. *J Parapsychol.* 2006;70(1):91-120.

341. Solfvin J, Roney-Dougal SM. A re-analysis and summary of data from a study of experienced versus novice yoga practitioners. In: Rao KR, ed. *Yoga and Parapsychology: Empirical Research and Theoretical Studies.* Delhi: Motilal Banarsidass; 2010.

342. Kolodziejzyk G. 2012; http://www.remote-viewing.com/, accessed March 30, 2012.

343. Schwartz S. *Opening to the Infinite.* Buda, TX: Nemoseen Media; 2007.

344. Kolodziejzyk G. Greg Kolodziejzyk's 13 year associative remote viewing experiment results. *J Parapsychol.* In press.

345. Myer-Czetli N. *Silent Witness: The Story of a Psychic Detective.* New York: Carol Pub. Group; 1993.

346. Yeterian D. *Casebook of a Psychic Detective.* New York: Stein and Day; 1982.

347. Leggett AJ. Macroscopic realism: What is it, and what do we know about it from experiment. In: Healey RA, Hellman G, eds. *Quantum Measurement: Beyond Paradox.* Minneapolis: University of Minnesota Press; 1998.

348. Reid MD. Incompatibility of macroscopic local realism with quantum mechanics in measurements with macroscopic uncertainties. *Phys Rev Lett.* March 27, 2000;84(13):2765-2769.

349. Groblacher S, Paterek T, Kaltenbaek R, et al. An experimental test of non-local realism. *Nature.* April 19, 2007;446(7138):871-875.

350. Scheidl T, Ursin R, Kofler J, et al. Violation of local realism with freedom of choice. *Proc Natl Acad Sci U S A.* November 16, 2010;107(46):19708-19713.

351. Walborn SP, Salles A, Gomes RM, Toscano F, Souto Ribeiro PH. Revealing hidden Einstein-Podolsky-Rosen nonlocality. *Phys Rev Lett.* April 1, 2011;106(13):130402.

352. Wheeler JA. Information, physics, quantum: The search for links. In: Zurek W, ed. *Complexity, Entropy, and the Physics of Information.* Reading, MA: Addison-Wesley; 1990.

353. Hoffman DD. Conscious realism and the mind-body problem. *Mind and Matter.* 2008;6(1):87-121.

354. Tressoldi PE, Storm L, Radin D. Extrasensory perception and quantum models of cognition. *NeuroQuantology.* 2010;8(4, Suppl 1):S81-87.

355. Anderson M. Is quantum mechanics controlling your thoughts? *Discover.* February 2009.

356. McAlpine K. Nature's hot green quantum computers revealed. *New Scientist.* February 3, 2010.

357. Ball P. Physics of life: The dawn of quantum biology. *Nature.* 2011;474:272-274.

358. Vedral V. Living in a quantum world. *Scientific American.* 2011:38-43.

359. Barreiro JT. Quantum physics: Environmental effects controlled. *Nature Physics.* 2011;7:927-928.

360. Walker EH. The quantum theory of psi phenomena. *Psychoenergetic Systems.* 1979;3:259-299.

361. Jahn RG, Dunne BJ. On the quantum mechanics of consciousness with application to anomalous phenomena. *Found Physics.* 1986;16:721-772.

362. Barnosky AD, Hadly EA, Bascompte J, et al. Approaching a state shift in Earth's biosphere. *Nature.* 2012;486(7401):52-58.

363. Abbasi K. Mass extinction of life is imminent. *J R Soc Med.* December 2010;103(12):471-472.

364. Laszlo E. *Quantum Shift in the Global Brain: How the New Scientific Reality Can Change Us and Our World.* Rochester, VT: Inner Traditions; 2008.

365. Laszlo E. *Science and the Akashic Field: An Integral Theory of Everything.* 2nd ed. Rochester, VT: Inner Traditions; 2007.

366. de Quincey C. *Consciousness from Zombies to Angels: The Shadow and the Light of Knowing Who You Are.* Rochester, VT: Park Street Press; 2009.

367. Skokowski P. I, zombie. *Conscious Cogn.* March 2002;11(1):1-9.

368. Mashour GA, LaRock E. Inverse zombies, anesthesia awareness, and the hard problem of unconsciousness. *Conscious Cogn.* December 2008;17(4):1163-1168.

369. Planck M. Consciousness matters. *The Observer.* January 25, 1931.

370. Pais A. *The Genius of Science: A Portrait Gallery.* Oxford, UK: Oxford University Press; 2000.

371. Linde A. Inflation, quantum cosmology and the anthropic principle. In: Barrow JD, Davies PCW, Jr. Harper CL, eds. *Science and Ultimate Reality: Quantum Theory, Cosmology and Complexity, Honoring John Wheeler's 80th Birthday.* Cambridge, UK: Cambridge University Press; 2004:451.

372. Wigner E. The unreasonable effectiveness of mathematics in the natural sciences. Richard Courant Lecture in Mathematical Sciences delivered at New York University, May 11, 1959. *Comm Pure Appl Math.* 1960;13(1).

373. Penrose R. What is reality? *New Scientist.* November 18, 2005.

374. Laszlo E. *Science and the Akashic Field.* Rochester, VT: Inner Traditions; 2004.

375. Radin D. Intention and reality: The ghost in the machine returns. *SHIFT: At the Frontiers of Consciousness.* Vol 15. Petaluma, CA: Institute of Noetic Sciences; 2007.

376. Dolan RM. *UFOs and the National Security State: Chronology of a Coverup, 1941–1973.* Charlottesville, VA: Hampton Roads; 2002.

377. Dolan RM. *The Cover-Up Exposed, 1973–1991 (UFOs and the National Security State, Vol. 2).* Rochester, NY: Keyhole Publishing; 2009.

378. Vallee J. *Wonders in the Sky: Unexplained Aerial Objects from Antiquity to Modern Times.* New York: Tarcher; 2010.

379. Story about an airship. *New York Times.* April 28, 1897.

380. Topics of the times. That mysterious airship. *New York Times.* March 19, 1987.

381. Jung CG. *Flying Saucers: A Modern Myth of Things Seen in the Skies.* London: Harcourt, Brace; 1959.

382. Thompson K. *Angels and Aliens.* New York: Ballantine Books; 1993.

383. Bullard TE. *The Myth and Mystery of UFOs*: Lawrence: University Press of Kansas; 2010.

384. Harman WW. *Global Mind Change: The Promise of the 21st Century.* San Francisco: Berrett-Koehler; 1998.

INDEX

INDEX

INDEX

INDEX

INDEX

Solar principle, 111
Solar system, 157, 313
Soma, 39
Southern Baptists, 19–20
Spielberg, Steven, 74
Spirits, discernment of, 63
Spiritual hedonism, 7
Spontaneous remissions, 60–61
Spoon bending, 219–220
Squires, Euan, 240
SRI International, 142
Sri Lanka, 55
Stanford University, 4, 311
Stanovich, Keith, 74–75, 77
Stapp, Henry, 240
Star Trek (television series), 70, 108
Stargate, 269
Sterling Hospital, Ahmedabad, India, 125, 126
Stevenson, Ian, 55, 56
Stimulants, 7
Stimulus-preceding negativity, 152
Stock market, 287–292
Storm, Lance, 195–196
Storr, Anthony, 5
Strassman, Rick, 36–37, 42–43
Strength building, 23
Stretching, 20, 23, 95
Subjective antedating, 157
Subtle energies, 319
Sufi rapid wound healing, 85
Summers, Montague, 63
Sunk cost bias, 82, 88
Superevidence, 136
Superior parietal lobe, 80
Superman (television show), xviii
Supernormal, coining of word, xviii–xix
Superstition, 1, 5, 9, 147–148, 310
Superstrength, 9, 110–111
Superstring theory, 270
Sutra, defined, 96
Swann, Ingo, 269
Swedish gymnastics, 24
Symbols, 310
Sympathetic nervous system, 148, 149, 207

Tantra (energy or kundalini), 22
Tantric sexual practices, 45
Tape delay, 157
Tart, Charles, 76
Taylor, Sam, 56

Telepathy, xxi, 1, 9, 77, 82–83, 84, 107–110, 127, 128, 129, 179–199, 205, 270, 276, 282
Bayesian analyses and, 197–198
brain scan tests and, 193–194
differed from clairvoyance, 268
example session, 186–188
ganzfeld, 128, 129, 184, 185–192, 194–198, 276
meta-analyses and, 196–197
multiple sessions, 188–190
noise reduction and, 194–196
skepticism and, 191–192, 196
tests outside laboratory, 199
Twain and, 180–181
Teresa, Saint, 62
Textbooks, psychology, 74–75, 77
Thaddeus, P., 244
Thailand, 55
Thalbourne, Michael, 89
Theosophical Society, 15, 270
Theosophist Magazine, 218
Theravada Buddhism, 53
Thinking-Feeling personality, 89
Thompson, Keith, 316
Tibet, 57
Time magazine, 20, 269–270
Time-reversed design, 166–167, 177, 263
Timelessness, 156
Tipitaka (Pali Canon), 53
TM-Sidhi program, 202–204, 215
Tobacco, 7
Tonglen meditation, 207
Tracks in the Psychic Wilderness (Graff), 272
Train Your Mind, Change Your Brain (Begley), 28
Transcendence, extreme sports and, 44–45
Transcendental Meditation (TM), 16, 17, 202–205
Transcranial magnetic or electrical stimulation, 7
Transiency, 51
Transliminality, 89
Tressoldi, Patrizio, 162–163, 165, 195–198
Tripartite philosophy, 307
Tucker, Jim, 55–56
Tulkus (reincarnated monks), 279
Tummo meditation, 123
Turkey, 55
Turning East (Cox), 17–18
Twain, Mark (Samuel Clemens), 180–181
Type 1 and 2 temperament, 228, 229

INDEX